RESCUE YOUR BACK

RESCUE YOUR BACK

A GUIDE FOR A NEW APPROACH TO BACK PAIN

CATHY MAHON, PT, MS

The Mahon Group, LLC
Annapolis, Maryland

Library of Congress Control Number: 2007012345

ISBN: 978-0-615-28069-1

Published by:
 The Mahon Group, LLC
1610 West Street
Suite 103
Annapolis, MD 21401
Telephone: 410-263-0333
www.TheMahonGroup.com

Editing by Elana Kann and Ron Kenner

Illustrations by Diane Abeloff and Joyce Hurwitz

Photographs by Frederick Soo

Cover Design by Elizabeth Tomlin

Layout Design by Jonathan Gullery

DVD Produced by E. Eric Johnson, III

(For contact information see Appendix D)

Printed in the United States of America

First Edition

Contents

To Richard — for being who you are

Please Read Before Using This Book

TERMS OF USE: This book contains information that is not intended to replace the services of trained health professionals or be a substitute for medical care. YOU ARE TO IMPLEMENT THIS PROGRAM WITH THE HELP OF A LICENSED PHYSICAL THERAPIST. This book is also designed for use in conjunction with the DVD or other materials with which it came packaged. If you choose to use this information, YOU AGREE to the terms contained herein. IF YOU DO NOT AGREE then return this book along with all materials to the publisher for a refund per our refund policy.

This book expresses the views and opinions of the Author. It does not necessarily express the views and opinions of the publisher. The information in this book is intended primarily as a means of creating awareness of an alternative approach to back pain and to provide guidelines to increase your potential for success. Every person is unique and the information presented may not be appropriate for your specific situation. So you are advised to seek the help of a licensed physical therapist to determine if this approach is appropriate for you. Therefore, of necessity, the publisher and author make no warranty of any kind, whether expressed or implied, and they will not be liable for any injury or harm you or others may suffer as a result of the use or attempted use of these materials, including but not limited to consequential, special, incidental, or punitive damages.

About The Author

CATHY Mahon, PT, MS has been practicing physical therapy for twenty-three years receiving a Master of Science Degree in Physical Therapy from Boston University in 1986 and a Bachelor of Science Degree in Kinesiology from the University of Maryland in 1983. She has acquired an expertise in orthopedics in the area of pain and dysfunction of the spine and extremities. At the time of this publication, Cathy continues to operate a private practice in Annapolis, Maryland which focuses on back pain.

Acknowledgments

WHEN I started writing this book I was under the impression it would take a year to complete. The book took over two and a half years. The last year and a half required a huge push. Needless to say, that didn't happen without a great deal of help from a number of wonderful and talented people.

This was very much a family project, so I would first like to thank my family, especially my husband Richard who did all the business side of publishing the book, picked up most of the family responsibilities, including all the brownie and cub scout meetings, kept a private practice going and was still there with a hug whenever I needed one. I want to thank my wonderful children, Cayla and Ryan for being who they are. It helped immensely to receive Cayla's notes and drawings full of love and encouragement and to see Ryan's six year old smiling face when he served us breakfast in bed. (The coffee has improved considerably over time.)

The most significant influence in my professional development has been my mother. She had an unparalleled ability to listen to people and connect with them. I could never thank her enough for her incredible example, as the first step in helping someone is to listen to them. I miss her greatly. At the same time my father contributed countless pearls of wisdom. When my brother was 25 he remarked that although our father didn't often give advice, when he did, did we ever know him to be wrong. His advice through the years has been invaluable and something I continually benefit from.

My brother Brad helped immensely to get this project started; and his two daughters, Michelle and Melissa have been close to us all along the way. Michelle has great insight, she made many suggestions and at one point helped to name the book. Melissa has continually supported us and provides a joy that is uniquely hers.

Also in my family are four people to whom I am extremely grateful. My brilliant and thoughtful nephew, Patrick, whose insights and suggestions contributed significantly. My beautiful nieces Elizabeth and Andrea modeled for the DVD and book. They worked long days and did a great job demonstrating what your back can do, whether it is good for your back or not. Fortunately for us Elizabeth is also an extremely talented graphic designer and created our book cover and DVD label. She also helped endlessly, contributing greatly during production of the DVD, and pitching in whenever she could. Last, but not least, thanks to Matt for patiently sharing Elizabeth with us.

There would not be a book if it were not for many people who entrusted me with their health. I have been blessed to work with truly amazing souls. I thank them for all they taught me and for the contribution they made towards the health and well being of others.

After my mother and father the key influences have been; Beverly Biondi PT, who jump started my journey when she recommended that before starting stabilization exercises that the physical therapist should make sure the patient has the necessary range of motion; Florence Kendell PT, who helped illustrate the effect of muscles on posture; Dr. Patricia Sullivan PT, who instructed therapeutic exercise emphasizing the need to structure and progress an exercise program based on the patient's ability. A special thanks to the family of the late Jim Gould from whom I learned so much in my early years. Thanks also to those who helped me secure a good foundation 24 years ago, Dr. Pam Levangie, Dr. Joyce White, Dr. Shirley Stockmeyer, Jim Porterfield, and Kate Schwartz. I would be amiss if I did not mention those who have significantly impacted the profession including, Dr. Stanley Paris, Dr. Geoffrey Maitland, Dr. Shirley Sahrmann, Dr. Julie Fritz, Dr. Anthony Delitto and the many professionals who work tirelessly at the American Physical Therapy Association and the World Confederation for Physical Therapy. Physical therapy has numerous professionals contributing constantly in many ways, it is impossible to mention them all, I apologize for those I have not mentioned.

I am deeply indebted to Elana Kann, my editor. She has practically lived with me for the past two years, at least inside my head. Elana gave so much of herself to organize an enormous amount of information, shaping it into the structured cohesive presentation that is now Rescue Your Back.

Then along came Ron Kenner, my polish editor and his assistant Tom Puckett. Ron's experience was helpful with different aspects of this project; his command over words helped the complicated matters flow a little easier.

I was also privileged to work with Diane Ableoff and Joyce Hurwitz, two extraordinary medical illustrators, who with the patience of Job agreed to work with a novice. They skillfully worked on all of my ideas and graciously gave me feedback as needed.

On this journey, we traveled to Seattle to film the DVD. Thanks to Eric Johnson at Lill Monster Motion Pictures and his wife Jen, it was a remarkable and memorable event. Eric is incredibly talented, having won multiple Emmy's and we were honored to have him help us with our project. He filmed an enormous amount of information in 3 days, creating a DVD that is extraordinarily helpful. While in Seattle we met Fred Soo, our still photographer. Fred had an unbelievable ability to capture the precise angles of our models for the still shots, which immeasurably contributed to the quality of the book.

Kelly Johnson has been a great friend and a key source of support and advice. She went so far as to alert me to new research and take care of my family's needs while we were making the DVD. I would be amiss if I didn't mention Kelly's children, Emma and Camille, who helped my children have a wonderful time in Seattle. We also enjoyed Seattle hospitality via Pam Deutsch and Ken Brettman who graciously let us stay at their home.

As the project neared its end, we have come to know Jonathan Gullery, Bob Powers and the staff at Books Just Books who have been simply wonderful. They have been tolerant of our many questions and lack of experience, helping us put together all the pieces of the puzzle to produce this book.

We were very fortunate to have the help of Chuck Tobin, Elisa Westapher and Robert Labate from Holland and Knight, LLP. They were incredibly responsive to my last minute needs with great interest and legal expertise.

All the while life went on at home. Thanks to some special people our life maintained a certain level of sanity. Linda Suskie and Ann Ward are two wonderful and gifted teachers who made it much easier to start this project knowing our children were in their capable hands. Cayla and Ryan have continued to have the support of outstanding teachers including, Kirsten Ernstes, Molly Gulden, Patricia Pumphrey, Katie Purfield, and Courtney Truntich. We are grateful to Kim Pletcher, the school counselor, for her sage words of advice. Finally, we are thankful for everyone at Lothian Elementary School for being the family that has supported our family during a very hectic time.

Along the way there have been many other people who have contributed to the accomplishment of this book, anywhere from an important word of advice to reviewing the manuscript. I want to thank; Mary Applegate, Chris Barry, Ellen Berry, Dr. Richard Bernstein, Dr. Christophe Boulay, Missy Cassidy, Luke Dreyer, Maureen Egen, Joyce Miller, Marilyn Higgs, Dwight Peters, Klara Ritsinias, Sandra Rogers, Dr. Shirley Sahrmann, Andrea Schoonover, Beth Smith, Linda Stuart, Karen Weed, Elsie Whitman, and Kim and Tad Woodward.

Last, but certainly not least, to a great group of people who provide perpetual support; Kelly Johnson, Laddie Franz, Chris Barry, Mike Dowling, Patrick Latham, Drew Loizeaux, Neil Levine, Joe Martin, Dan Nissenbaum and Bob Blongiewicz.

A Personal Note from the Author

THIS book seeks to improve back pain evaluation and treatment by providing an alternative approach; one that opens up a whole new avenue to explore what is happening to your body and causing your pain.

The major challenge and a fundamental problem in the treatment of back pain is that 85 percent of the time the cause is unknown;[1] obviously it is difficult to treat something when you do not know the cause. This book presents a basic, straight-forward approach that I believe can identify the cause of back pain for many people.

Following is the fundamental point of this book.

In October 2007 the publication, Diagnosis and Treatment of Low Back Pain: A Joint Clinical Practice Guideline from the American College of Physicians and the American Pain Society, confirmed that, of those who see their primary care physician, for more than 85 percent of the cases the cause of back pain is unknown.[2]

As a society we have to ask ourselves the obvious question: **What is missing?** I believe we've been focusing on problems in the back for so long that we have missed the problems in our bodies—***other than*** the back—that cause back pain.

The approach presented in this book not only asks whether you have back problems, it also asks whether your back is having body problems.

This approach takes some of the basic measurements physical therapists learn in school a few steps further to explore whether there is a relationship between the description of your pain and limitations in mechanics throughout your body.

To find time to write this book I have not scheduled many new patients for two and a half years. As I was putting my thoughts together, I was interested in the patients' opinions of this evaluation and treatment. An informal, anonymous survey was sent to the last fifty patients who had this evaluation and who developed an initial home exercise program. Although I expected to hear some positive responses, I found the feedback quite remarkable.

- 100 percent of the respondents said the evaluation was effective in helping them under-stand their pain.

- 100 percent of the respondents said the program to manage their pain on a daily basis was effective.

- 100 percent said the exercise program to address their limitations was effective.

- More than 85 percent of the respondents gave the highest rating of "very effective" to all three of these areas.

Some of you might ask why I wrote this for you instead of for health care providers. My response is that information moves slowly through the health care system and many aspects of health care have developed into quite a large industry. It could take years for me to get the information through the industry to a physical therapist (PT) near you. The alternative is to inform you, so that you can ask a PT in your area to work with you on this approach to your back pain.

I also wrote this book for you because you have a great deal of power. Given that we live in a consumer-driven world, you have the power to go to a PT and the clinic administrator and request the time to do this evaluation and the one-on-one time with the PT for follow-up sessions. As a consumer, you also have the power to influence your insurance company. That is not to say it will be easy. However, making a well-thought-out request can be helpful for you and if enough people make the same request that will most definitely have an effect. Finally, with the information from the book and the results of your evaluation, you have the power to make changes in your life to improve the health of your body.

I truly believe that this approach is the missing link in the treatment for many people with back pain. At the same time, for your success you need to be aware of the challenges you face. Back pain is an enormous subject matter and I do not have all of the answers.

Two of the goals of this book are to stimulate research and to promote an exchange of ideas. Do not wait until the research is in. You could be waiting a long time. Instead, pursue the evaluation. For many of you the evaluation will reveal, very clearly, the limitations in your body that affect your back. Then work with your PT on what you can do *now* for your back pain.

This book focuses on the basic information, including an outline of the evaluation and treatment. The outline is meant to serve as a guide for you as you work with your PT. I hope I achieved a balance in providing enough information to be helpful and in keeping it short enough to be manageable. I welcome your feedback to my website.

CHAPTER 1

About this Approach

WHY THIS BOOK?

A **YOUNG** man came in for a physical therapy evaluation; he barely complained about his pain. He had seen two very good clinicians about his back pain, but was still having trouble. The evaluation of his mechanics revealed extensive mechanical limitations throughout his body including significant limitations in flexibility. His back demonstrated good movement which was clearly one of the only places he could move from to perform many activities. Since his back was compensating for so many limitations, I wondered why he did not complain about more back pain. Although work interfered a little with his ability to follow through on the exercise program, he improved. A month after he started therapy he reported that he was much better. He also said that when he first started therapy he was so bothered by the pain that he felt suicidal. This experience was a significant influence on my motivation to write this book. Long before he acknowledged the full extent of his problems, the measurements accurately and clearly revealed how extensive his problems were.

Another patient, a very intelligent woman, worked extraordinarily hard to avoid surgery but was unable to do so. She came to my office after she had back surgery. During the evaluation she could feel and see the limitations in her mechanics. She reported being previously completely unaware of these limitations. We discussed how these limitations impacted her back during activity. She wondered whether she could have avoided the surgery if she'd had this evaluation before the surgery. Her experience parallels a number of other patients. There are times when surgery or other invasive treatment cannot be avoided. However, her story illustrates the desire people have to try and improve their health *before* undergoing more invasive treatment.

The knee is a simpler environment to demonstrate the link between pain, limitations, and wear and tear on a joint. A 23-year-old with a history of five knee surgeries, three to reconstruct her knee, was once again experiencing pain along with increased difficulty walking. The evaluation of her mechanics revealed a significant loss of motion in her ankle joint as well as limitations in her hip and upper body. When she focused on increasing the motion in her ankle her pain decreased and her walking significantly improved. I spoke to her a year and a half later and she said it had been the longest period of time that she had gone without a surgery. Her knee felt better and she had even started running.

I believe that the loss of range of motion in her ankle had forced her knee to be positioned poorly during activity. That caused the pain and the repeated wear and tear on her knee joint.

If you picked up this book you probably already realize that the treatment of back pain is a great challenge to our society. Open any book about back pain and you are likely to find a comment about the millions of people who have back pain and also a remark about the difficulty we have treating it. When you have back pain I believe you have two problems: 1) the cause of your back pain, and 2) access to care.

I believe this approach should be one of the first steps when trying to identify the cause of back pain, or any joint pain. This doesn't mean that mechanical limitations are the cause of *all* pain. It means that whenever dealing with back or body pain it is important to look at the body as a system and determine if there are limitations in the body that are contributing to the pain.

Regarding the second problem, I received some feedback recommending that I not discuss the challenges in accessing care. Comments were made along the lines of, people don't want to hear that, people just want to know whether this approach will work for them, or, from a marketing stand point, keep it positive. I completely believe in this approach and could easily write a book solely about this approach and it would paint a very positive picture. With the great number of people who have back pain I would likely sell a good many books. However, I believe it will greatly increase the chance that you will be successful if you know the challenges you face, with both the approach and accessing care. I am not focused on selling books, rather I am working to help as many people as possible by increasing awareness that there is an alternative approach to back pain for many of you, and to make you aware of the challenges you face. If I do not discuss the second problem I would only be helping you with one of your two problems.

So here we go. There are two parts to the problem of accessing care: 1) finding a professional with the knowledge of the treatment you need, and 2) the money to pay for the treatment. The approach in this book will help address the knowledge issue for those of you with limitations in your body that cause your back pain, those for whom this book is written. So for you, the primary issue to accessing care is money.

On one hand the issue is simple; I believe that many PTs would offer this approach if they knew they could put food on their table, pay their staff and keep the doors of their office open. If the PT is reimbursed for her/his time your access to this approach would significantly improve. However on the other hand, the present system of reimbursement is complex and convoluted. To say it poses a huge problem for physical therapists is an understatement.

My hope is that many of you will ask a PT to help you with this approach and call your insurance company to approve the treatment. Some of you may not have trouble finding a PT and having your insurance company agree to pay for the treatment. However, many of you will be pioneers. You will have to work to convince a clinic in your area to help you with this approach. You might also need to work with your insurance company to present your case as to why this approach is in the best interest of both you and the insurance company.

Here is some information you can take with you. Recent research concludes:

- Exercise was found to be an effective intervention for prevention of BP's, (back problems.) [3]

- Surgery only marginally improves the quality of life for those with chronic low back pain. [4]

- Medicare expenditures for back pain increased 629 percent in epidural steroid injections, [5] the number of MRI's increased for Medicare beneficiaries 307 percent, [6] and the number of spinal fusion surgeries increased 220 percent. [7] At the same time there was not a decrease in the number social security disability recipients. [8, 9]

- 85 percent of patients have non-specific low back pain which means the cause of their pain is unknown. [10]

In addition you can inform the PT or the insurance officials of the advantages you read about in this book. For example, this approach is based on objective data: the measurements of your body. The data are compared to a detailed, objective and measurable description of your pain. Your progress is reassessed with objective measures that are tailored to you. They might also be interested to know that there is a Quick Relief Strategy for you to learn to decrease your pain on your own and that a significant amount of the treatment program is designed for you to do at home, both decreasing the number of visits to a clinician.

So, Why this book? I wrote this book as the best avenue to move people in a new direction. I also thought this was the best avenue to stimulate research, to promote discussion and to increase each individual's chance of being successful with this approach. I hope the book creates a stir and gains enough attention that your efforts will pave the way for those who follow.

Initially I was more tempered in my comments. Then I realized that this is my opportunity to inform and inspire you. I have been a physical therapist for twenty three years. I have seen and learned a great deal; for several years I worked as a traveling physical therapist and then I worked in my home state filling in as a temporary PT in many different physical therapy offices. Combined I had the opportunity to work in over forty clinics.

Eventually, I started my own practice. I live in a state where I do not have to rely on physicians to refer patients and I do not participate with insurance companies. (My patients submit their bills to get the reimbursement.) I can focus my energy on the patient. We both work hard and it has proven successful for many patients.

I hope that one day this approach will move into the mainstream and become easily accessible to help as many people as possible.

THE SYSTEM LIMITATIONS APPROACH TO PAIN

This book presents the System Limitations Approach to Pain™ (SLAP). SLAP is based on the theory that your body works as an integrated system and that limitations in one physical location in the system can cause problems that place excess force on another physical location in the system. This can result in pain and wear and tear in that area of the body.

The limitations that SLAP focuses on are limitations in your mechanics. The foundation of SLAP is that your back pain is a result of excess force placed on your back; either from your back compensating for mechanical limitations or from being poorly positioned due to mechanical limitations. The stories that follow are provided to help you understand a little more about this approach.

Consider the following: You have five employees working on a project designed to have all of them participate. If two are not doing their job, the other three are left to do all of the work. The three employees, doing more work than originally designed for them, eventually get tired, angry, and break down. The two who are not doing the job designed for them do not get tired, angry, or break down. You might need to directly help the three employees if they are injured. *However, the two who are not doing their jobs are the real underlying problem.* This story demonstrates that the physical location of pain does not always reveal the actual source of the underlying problem.

This lesson applies to mechanics in the body. Two joints serve to open and close your mouth when you talk and eat. If the joint on the right side of your mouth has a mechanical limitation such as decreased range of motion, the joint on the left substitutes by providing more motion than it was originally designed for to open your mouth to talk and to eat. As a result of the increased activity, the left side will start to hurt. Later an x-ray might show the left joint wearing down from the increased activity, and eventually you might need to have a surgical reconstruction to repair the left joint. If the reconstruction is done and the decreased range of motion persists in the right joint, the reconstruction of the left joint will also suffer the same extra force and activity that wore the left joint down to begin with, in which case the reconstruction might start to wear down, too. In this instance the limited range of motion in the right joint *is the real underlying problem* that needs to be addressed to adequately treat your left joint problems.

Now apply that lesson to your back pain. In this theory you can have limitations in the mechanics in your body, such as loss of range of motion or strength in your arms, legs, or trunk; and, just like the two employees not doing their job, the limitations in your mechanics can force your back to perform activity that your back is not designed for. When your back performs this activity over and over again during daily activities, it can lead to pain as well as wear and tear on your spine. *In this case, specific mechanical limitations in your body, other than your back, are the underlying problem for the back pain* and are critical to address for the successful treatment of your back pain.

There are other approaches that might sound similar to this approach as their intention is to address your physical body; however, five points distinguish this approach to pain.

1) LIMITATIONS

A large number of people, including clinicians, are unaware of the significant limitations many have in the mechanics required for basic everyday activities such as standing, walking, sitting, and lying down. You and your clinician might think you are using poor posture or poor body mechanics and that you simply need to pay more attention and use better posture. In the SLAP approach, you learn whether limitations in your mechanics make it *impossible* to use good posture and good body mechanics in the activities that increase your pain.

Most of you have certain activities that repeatedly cause your pain. Unaware of your mechanical limitations, many continue to perform those activities. With back pain it is usually your back that is substituting for the limitations in your mechanics, during those activities. This places extra force on your back and it is this force, I believe, that causes your back pain.

2) SYSTEM

Another aspect that distinguishes this approach is the realization that limitations can be located anywhere in the body and still be directly related to the position of your back and its subsequent pain. The System Limitations Approach to Pain assumes that your body works as one system. In SLAP the PT will look for limitations in your mechanics, from your head to your toe, related to:

- the specific positions of your back that increase your pain
- the activities in your life that increase your pain

3) SPECIFIC

You want to be very specific about what to address. When tuning a guitar you cannot just tighten any string; rather, you tighten a certain string and tighten it a specific amount. Many programs that publicize helping with back pain will identify changes in your body and recommend some type of stretching, strengthening, stabilization, posture or massage. When mechanical limitations affect your back, it is not helpful to do simply any exercise or massage type of work. In this approach, measuring your limitations and determining how they are specifically related to the activities and positions of your back that increase your back pain is the *unique step* that allows you to develop a program tailored to your needs. The beauty of the *specific measurements* is that you determine what to specifically address.

You also need to be *very specific* in your description of pain. Use frequency, intensity and duration to help you describe your pain in specific terms. The more specific you are the more you can learn about your back pain and the better choices you will make during the development of your program.

4) PAIN

In the SLAP approach, pain is not considered the problem. We cannot peel back your skin and look to see what is happening inside your back; we cannot see what the joints, muscles, and nerves are doing during your activities. In this approach, we use your pain as a reporter from inside your body to teach us all it can about how your tissue is responding to positions and activities. The pain and symptoms will serve as your guide to protect your back and help design your exercise program.

In this book, the terms "your pain" or "your back pain" refer to any of the pain or symptoms that are a part of your back problems. This includes pain, numbness, or changes in sensation anywhere in your back, arms or legs. While this book focuses on low back pain, the information applies to the whole back.

5) APPROACH

This is an approach, not a method. The beginning and end are not the same for everyone. Guidelines are provided to start to approach your back pain; however your individual situation is what directs the development of your program. This approach teases out your unique problems and addresses them rather than conforming you to a program that possesses its own agenda. You and your PT approach your back pain based on information about *your* pain, *your* mechanical limitations, and *your* activities.

EVALUATION AND TREATMENT IN SLAP

The initial evaluation in SLAP is the easy part. It focuses on identifying your basic mechanical limitations whether they contribute a little or a lot to what is causing your pain. Many of you will need a more detailed evaluation in certain areas and your PT will use several sources to help identify those areas including; information from the initial evaluation, your response to treatment, the pain that persists, and information from the re-evaluation.

When the evaluation reveals that mechanical limitations are causing your back pain, the next step is to develop your program. Developing the program to address your limitations and protect your back is much more challenging than the evaluation itself. Improving your mechanics is not easy. Presently there is little research on how to change our bodies' mechanics. The hope is that research will be helpful in finding the quickest, most effective means to improve mechanics. Research will take a long time. Meanwhile the specific measurements and specific details about the nature of your pain can guide the development of your program.

The goal is to minimize the forces on your body that cause pain and wear and tear on your back. You will address all of your mechanical limitations in order to move your body as close as possible to ideal mechanics.

Some of you have mechanical limitations that are fairly easy to address. Others have mechanical limitations and combinations of limitations that are more difficult to address. In either case, the more you know about your pain the better decisions you can make.

OVERVIEW OF THIS APPROACH

This section provides an overall view of how this approach is ordered. As you progress through the book, pieces will be filled in. Refer back to this section as needed.

Although you are integral to the success of your evaluation and treatment, to adequately identify your mechanical limitations and their relationship to your pain you do need to partner with a physical therapist (PT). In this approach, your PT evaluates the most basic mechanics throughout your body that impact your back and helps you develop your treatment programs. Please do not be lured by a well-meaning friend who wants to help you with this approach, regardless of his or her health care background. Improving your mechanics while protecting your back is not quick and easy. Physical therapists are uniquely qualified to provide this approach.

EVALUATION

In this approach you spend much time with your PT in the beginning for your evaluation and for the follow-up sessions to develop your program. It takes time to do the evaluation. The PT listens to your description of the pain, facilitates writing an objective and measurable description, takes the measurements, and explains the findings. If mechanical limitations are related to your pain, it takes additional time to teach you the initial steps necessary to protect your back.

While the name of the evaluation for SLAP is the System Limitations Evaluation, with back pain the evaluation is the System Limitations Evaluation for Back Pain. The most critical parts of the evaluation are:

1. History: your experience with pain described in objective, detailed, measurable terms. This is the time to discuss any other medical history with your PT.

2. Measurements: the PT takes measurements to identify if there are mechanical limitations. The PT provides any other tests or measurements indicated.

3. Assessment: the PT determines whether there is a relationship between the limitations identified in your mechanics and the description of your pain.

4. Plan: the PT plans the development of your Protective and Corrective Programs and any manual therapy your PT determines you need in order to make progress.

TREATMENT

Once your PT determines that mechanical limitations are causing your pain, you and your PT develop two programs to *rescue your back*. These are your Protective Program and your Corrective Program. You carry out the programs at home. The PT sessions are for developing your individual programs and for any manual physical therapy required to facilitate progress.

Your Protective Program has two parts. One is the plan for protecting your back during your daily activities. The other is a Quick-Relief Strategy, which consists of positions and techniques you can use to decrease your pain on your own. Chapter 5 includes blank pages for you to write down the information for your protective program. Writing it down helps to develop the program, creates a written record, tracks progress for motivation and program development, and increases your understanding of what is happening to your body. You can create a Protective Program Manual of your information.

The Corrective Program is the exercise program designed to address your mechanical limitations. Note the word here is "address"; I do not believe that we have the answers to correct all mechanical limitations. Also, many of us have never had ideal postural alignment or full range of motion and strength to begin with. The current goal of the Corrective Program is to move you as close to ideal mechanics as possible to protect your joints and the health of your body, thereby decreasing your pain and increasing your tolerance to activity. Work with your PT to set realistic goals to meet your potential. The first Corrective Program you develop will be termed your Initial Corrective Program. As you continue, your Corrective Program will progress accordingly.

Manual therapy is a hands-on treatment the PT directly applies to your body. I believe that most of your improvements result from improving your mechanics. Some of your progress will require manual therapy. I do not recommend manual therapy simply directed to decrease pain; rather I believe this therapy best serves to address the underlying mechanical limitations causing the pain and thereby decrease the pain.

INDEPENDENT MANAGEMENT

After you develop your Protective Program, develop your Initial Corrective Program, and demonstrate an ability to manage your pain on your own, many of you will go out and work independently for several weeks. After working on your own you will return to your PT to assess your status, address any problems, and progress your program.

The length of time you work on your own and the number of visits you have when you return depends on how significant your problems are and on your ability to independently manage your pain. Some of you might not go out on your own and instead will continue with PT sessions for manual therapy to facilitate your progress.

How many times you go through the cycle of working on your own and returning to your PT depends on how involved your pain and mechanical limitations are. Some of you might return only one time, while others of you who have had limitations for years or decades might return repeatedly for several years to progress your program.

IMPORTANT

I strongly recommend that you continue with your PT until you meet the goals you set with your PT. There is a big temptation for people to continue with their program and PT only while they have pain; once the pain is gone so is the program. But not surprisingly, without staying with the program and adequate attention to the problem the pain is likely to come back.

CHAPTER 2

Getting Started

Is This Approach For You?

THIS approach is for people who have mechanical limitations that are causing their back pain. The answer as to whether this approach is for you depends on other factors as well. When mechanical limitations are the greatest contributor to your back pain, I find that the single most important factor in your success is your attitude. Following are some thoughts to help you shape a successful attitude.

For most of you, your mechanical limitations did not originate in the past few months. They have been there for years or decades, and they are not going to go away in the next 6 months.

Most of us accept that it is going to take 3-5 years to pay for a car and 15-30 years to pay for a house. We also accept that we need a job 8 hours a day to make the money to pay for those things. However, despite the fact that our body is the only vehicle we get to take us through life most of us do not accept that our body requires time too.

The work to develop your treatment program reminds me of a roller coaster. The cart works for every inch in its climb up the first hill. Once it reaches a certain point the rest of the journey is much easier, although with its ups and downs. In the beginning you feel like you work for every inch of progress to understand what is going on with your body and to develop your protective and corrective programs. Once the programs are developed, the rest of the journey is much easier, although you still have your ups and downs.

Desiring a quick fix is not just a problem for an individual; it is a greater problem that is perpetuated by our society. We need to change the general understanding about pain and immediate gratification or the quick fix. If the quick fixes worked, back pain would not be the problem it is today.

These thoughts help shape a successful attitude towards your program, your daily expectations and your long term goals. If you have mechanical limitations that are causing your pain and you want a quick fix, or you want someone else to fix you, then this approach might not be successful for you; even though it might be what your physical body needs.

In that case I strongly recommend that you keep an open mind, read everything and possibly try this approach with a physical therapist who will work to help you gain an understanding about what is happening to your body. If you choose to try another approach first, then please keep these ideas in the back of your mind. If you then continue to have problems I hope you will return to pursue this approach at that time.

GENERAL FRAMEWORK OF INFORMATION IN THIS BOOK

THE REMAINDER OF CHAPTER 2 explains how to customize the book's information according to your pain and your activity level.

CHAPTER 3 describes the roles of pain, defines the Big Four Mechanics and Limitations, and explains how your back compensates for limitations in your mechanics.

CHAPTERS 4, 5, 6, AND 7 present the outline of the evaluation, protective program and corrective program. These outlines serve as a guide for you as you work with your PT.

CHAPTER 4 describes the System Limitations Evaluation to increase your understanding of this approach, to help you know what to expect, and to help you sort out whether the evaluation you receive is what this approach recommends. *Please review this chapter prior to going for your physical therapy evaluation.*

CHAPTER 5 explains the Protective Program. The Protective Program has two parts. One is the plan for how to protect your back during daily activities, and the other is a Quick Relief Strategy for you to be able to decrease your pain on your own. This chapter includes charts and boxes for you to write down your information. You can copy these pages and put them together to create a Protective Program Manual.

CHAPTER 6 introduces the Corrective Program. This chapter covers how to develop and progress the exercise program needed to address your mechanical limitations.

CHAPTER 7 contains exercises as examples of how to apply the exercise principles. I also include the exercises in case you and your PT want to consider some of these for your program.

CHAPTER 8 discusses the challenges to current treatment and how this approach addresses some of those challenges.

THE DVD demonstrates some ideas that are difficult to communicate solely on paper, including:

from Chapter 5, finding your best and worst back positions and planning helpful positions; and from Chapter 7, many of the exercises are demonstrated. The DVD is in a pocket at the back of this book.

Customizing This Book to Your Needs:
RED, YELLOW, or GREEN

People have different levels of back pain and different levels of problems performing activities. Some of you have only slight pain and some of you have severe pain. All of you are in the same group of back pain. I want all of you to read the whole book. There is a lot of information and so I want to help you identify where it is best to concentrate your energy as you get started. Based on your pain and activity level, three subgroups are defined to help you learn what information is most important to you. Although they are subgroups they will simply be referred to as groups. These groups are based on the frequency, intensity, and duration of your pain and your ability to perform daily functional activities. I believe that research will find that these groups are also related to the severity of the mechanical limitations. The greater your limitations the more likely you are in the YELLOW or RED group. The fewer limitations you have, the more likely you are in the GREEN group.

The groups are: RED = the most involved, this group has the most pain and most limitations in activities; YELLOW = the group in-between that has pain and limitations that are less disruptive than for the RED group; and GREEN = the least involved, this group has the least pain and fewest limitations in activities.

Each group participates in the whole program which includes the evaluation and the two treatment programs. Which group you are in affects *how you will move through* the program. For example, if you are in the GREEN group you might have the whole evaluation with all the tests and measurements in one appointment, while those of you in the RED group will not tolerate some of the tests for a long time. The RED group takes considerable time to develop a corrective program, while the GREEN group and some in the YELLOW will very quickly develop the exercises for the Initial Corrective Program.

Decide which group most closely resembles you. Keep in mind that there are millions of you in each group. The group description covers a *range* of experiences and is not a *specific description* of any one person's issues. Do not be concerned about information in the description that is not applicable to you. Your PT is there to make the changes to meet your needs. If you feel you are between groups, choose to follow the advice for the group that is more involved.

After you start, if you struggle to get control over your pain, if the exercises are difficult or your symptoms increase, talk to your physical therapist and re-think what group you are in. You might need to move to a more involved group and start using the information from that perspective.

The description of each group revolves around the frequency, intensity and duration of pain. The intensity of pain is based on a pain scale of 0-10. 0/10 represents no pain and 10/10 represents the worst pain you could have. The ranges of intensity of pain in the following descriptions are there as a guideline. A range is offered for each group because there are millions of you in each group and because one person's 6/10 could be another person's 4/10. In this approach the most important aspect of identifying your intensity level is to be consistent *with yourself* each time you use the scale, so that you can track your own progress.

DESCRIPTION AND READING GUIDE

Following is a description of each group and a reading guide. The reading guide is provided to try to make the book as reader friendly as possible. Based on which group you most closely resemble, the reading guide makes suggestions about where you should initially focus your energy. Again you should read the whole book and do the whole program with a PT. However there is a lot of information here and this section tries to customize the information so you can focus on the parts that are important to you as you move through your program.

RED GROUP

Description of RED:

The general frequency, intensity and duration for the RED group is pain that occurs daily for more than 60% of the day, pain that can be as low as 0/10, however most days will increase to above a 5/10 and pain that lasts anywhere from 20 minutes to all day.

Following is the general nature of pain and activity for the RED group.
Pain can increase with some or all of the following:

- Some light household chores such as dusting, folding laundry, pouring a drink.
- Most moderate and heavy household chores.
- Self-care including dressing, bathing, and grooming.
- Functional activities for less than 30 minutes such as sitting, standing, lying down, walking or driving.
- Walking up or down stairs or getting in or out of a car.

Which activity increases your pain is specific to you. Some of you might wake up at night several times because of the pain, while others find that lying down provides relief and therefore the pain does not wake you up at night.

In the RED group, pain increases during the day. The increase can occur as pain that progressively increases throughout the day resulting in pain from a 5/10 to a 10/10. Or the increase in pain can fluctuate. For example you are sitting and the pain increases to a 6/10; when you change position the pain subsides; then you are sitting again and the pain increases to a 6/10; when you change position the pain subsides.

Most days are disrupted by the pain. Your days could be disrupted during one or all of the following: your self-care activities such as dressing, bathing, grooming, light household chores, tasks at work, or social activities. On some days they could all be affected and on some days only one or two activities could be affected.

The pain is rarely a 0/10. If you are fortunate enough to have a position that decreases your pain, it is either limited to a certain period of time and then you need to change that position, or you have relief only as long as you are in the position and a brief time afterwards.

If you have tried different approaches to decrease your pain, they might have helped a little. If they helped a lot it was only temporary.

Some of you belong in the RED group not because of the intensity of your pain but because you have pain in multiple locations—shoulder, neck, hip, and back—and therefore learning how to manage your pain and developing a Protective Program will require as much time and effort as for someone who has more intense and frequent back pain.

Customizing Chapters for RED:

RED: Study Chapter 3, Back Pain and Basic Human Mechanics.

RED: Study Chapter 4, The System Limitations Evaluation, and seek out a physical therapist for your evaluation. When you are reading Chapter 4, the following will help you decide what to concentrate on:

- *History:* If you have had back pain for a long time or if you have additional areas of pain such as shoulder, neck, or leg pain, you might spend 50-60 minutes reporting your history to your PT. Your experience with pain is very important, so be as detailed, objective and measurable as you can be. For help to objectively describe your experience in detail, fill out as much as you can of Step 1 in Chapter 5, prior to your evaluation. With this level of pain life is usually quite difficult. Avoid the temptation to digress and discuss unrelated problems at work and home; your PT has a lot to take in, try to stay focused on you and your experience with the pain.
- *Posture Evaluation:* This is the first step in the physical evaluation. Some of you in the RED group might not be able to stand well or long enough for the full posture evaluation.
- *Range of Motion Evaluation:* Many of you will tolerate over half of the range of motion (ROM) evaluation. However, a number of you are in so much pain that your PT will have to judge

your limitations by your posture and by observing your movement. Your PT will then start teaching you your Protective Program to help you protect your back and to decrease your pain so eventually you will tolerate the remainder of your range of motion evaluation.

- *Motor Control Evaluation:* For most of you, your ability to control your back can be assessed over the first few sessions.
- *Strength Evaluation (Manual Muscle Test, or MMT):* Your initial evaluation will not include the strength test because your pain level suggests that your body is too fragile to tolerate this test. Also your pain would influence the test results. When you can safely have the strength evaluation depends on your individual situation. For some of you it could be more than 12 months before you safely tolerate it. There are some cases when the body is so fragile and the spine so compromised that a manual muscle test will never be tolerated.
- *Re-evaluation:* The re-evaluation of your measurements will not include a full re-test because most of you are trying to keep your pain down long enough to start the exercises in the Corrective Program. A complete re-test could be counterproductive. You might have re-measurements of a few areas to see how things are going, but not at the risk of losing the progress you have fought so hard for. Once you are feeling better you should have a re-evaluation of your measurements every 12 weeks. Occasionally a few measurements might be taken at 6 or 8 weeks, but that is rarely the case.

RED: Study Chapter 5, Your Protective Program. The initial focus for the RED group is the Protective Program. In the beginning you need to learn about the nature of your pain. Then you develop a program that helps you learn how to move through your day performing activities in a manner that protects your back and decreases your pain. For many of you the initial development of the program will take a concentrated effort.

In this group you will spend months developing a protective program. Initially to learn how to perform your daily activities in a manner that protects your back and decreases your pain. Then you will start to develop ways to perform activities you have not been able to do because of the pain.

Do as much of the first step in this chapter as possible before your PT evaluation. The PT will work on all the other steps in this chapter with you.

RED: Study Chapter 6, Your Corrective Program. For those of you in the RED group, the first week to a month you might use only a few carefully selected exercises from your Corrective Program, chosen for how well they decrease your pain. Your PT will then carefully progress your exercise program to address your mechanical limitations.

- *Range of Motion:* Your PT might choose stretching exercises that you can start in the first few weeks to decrease your pain; these exercises will become your Quick Relief Strategy. For the most involved people in the RED group the PT might have to help perform the stretches until enough progress is made and the stretches can be done independently. For those of you closer to the YELLOW group, you might complete your initial stretching program in 8 weeks.

- *Motor Control:* Many of you might tolerate the first motor control exercise recommended, once you can get into and out of the position. Usually the first position is on your back on the floor, because the exercise requires a surface firmer than a bed.
- *Strengthening:* Tolerance to strength training depends on a number of factors including your tolerance of the positions in which you exercise. Because of your pain and limitations you will most likely start strengthening before you ever tolerate the strength testing.
- *Posture:* Begin to work on improving postural alignment only after measurements show improvement in your range of motion. Efforts to improve alignment before you have improved mechanics can be very aggravating to your back.

People in the RED group are quite varied. Some of you might be ready for a full range of motion program in 8 weeks. Others of you will struggle to find positions that protect your back, in which case it could be 6-12 months before you have a full program for ROM. As soon as you can, start the first motor control exercise and abdominal strengthening (isometrics), so that you can increase your ability to control and coordinate your back position.

RED: Study Chapter 7, Exercises. You can use this chapter to reinforce your exercise technique for exercises that your PT selects for you. You can use the DVD as well for those specific exercises. When your PT needs to modify any of your exercises listen to your PT's instructions and not the book or DVD instructions.

YELLOW GROUP

Description of YELLOW:

The frequency, intensity, and duration for the YELLOW group vary significantly. In frequency your pain might be daily, weekly, monthly, yearly, or seasonal. Weekly pain means that while you have pain every week, there are days during the week when you are pain-free. In the monthly, yearly or seasonal patterns you have weeks or months of being close to pain-free, but when the pain comes on you alter your life to recover. This can happen in the spring when you start gardening, over the busy holiday time, or every few months or years depending on what is happening in your life.

The intensity of your pain is generally from a 0/10 - 6/10. Your pain can spike to a 7/10 - 10/10 because of specific activities or a series of activities. The pain does not usually go above a 6/10 every day. If your pain does go above a 6/10 every day, you might actually be more consistent with problems for the RED group. You fit with the YELLOW group only if the reason the pain increases above a 6/10 is very heavy labor, and if on the days you do not do heavy labor your pain decreases to a low intensity.

The duration varies too. A person in the YELLOW group can have pain every day all day long for months. Pain that lasts longer is a lower intensity such as a 1/10 to a 3/10. This pain can disrupt you but not stop you from your daily activities like self-care, getting in and out of bed, cooking, sitting for meals, doing light to moderate household chores. Pain that is of shorter duration, either a few hours or all day for a few days would be much more intense and require that you alter your daily activities to recover. In contrast, in the GREEN group the short duration pain would not alter basic daily activities; it might only affect heavy activity such as shoveling after a heavy snow storm.

Following is the general nature of pain and activity for the YELLOW group.
Pain can increase with some or all of the following:

- Light household chores if the position is one that increases your pain and is performed for a prolonged period of time.
- Moderate and heavy household chores such as washing dishes, pulling wet laundry out of the washing machine, and vacuuming.
- Prolonged functional activity such as sitting, standing, or walking for more than 30 minutes.
- Walking up or down stairs, or getting in or out of a car.

In the YELLOW group, most days you can do many mild-to-moderate household chores or work-related activities, but even though you do them, some can be painful. Pain is disruptive to your life, although you can have long periods throughout the day or week without much pain while doing quite a bit of activity. At times you have to choose activities wisely in order to control your pain. This could mean you have to consider things like the type of activity or the amount of time you participate in the activity.

The difference between the YELLOW and the GREEN group is that pain for those in the YELLOW group occurs more often and is more intense during daily activities such as self care, light to moderate house-hold chores, and functional activities such as sitting and standing. The difference between YELLOW and RED is that although the YELLOW group has pain they can still complete most daily activities, and they have longer periods of pain-free time.

Customizing Chapters for YELLOW:

YELLOW: Study Chapter 3, Back Pain and Basic Human Mechanics.

YELLOW: Study Chapter 4, System Limitations Evaluation, and seek out a physical therapist for your evaluation. The following will help you decide what information to concentrate on:

- *History:* Provide as detailed, measurable, and objective a description as possible. Work on the first step of the Protective Program and bring your written information to the evaluation.
- *Postural Evaluation:* Most of you will tolerate the entire postural evaluation.

- *Range of Motion Evaluation:* Most of you will have the entire range of motion evaluation.
- *Motor Control Evaluation:* Many of you will be assessed in the first session for your ability to control your back. Your PT will be able to get a sense of your trunk control through your posture and how you can hold your trunk when trying the first motor control exercise.
- *Strength Evaluation (Manual Muscle Test, or MMT):* You will not have the strength test during your initial evaluation. Those of you closer to the GREEN group might need to wait only a month or two, until the PT knows your body well enough to decide when it is appropriate for you to have the strength test.
- *Re-evaluation:* What will be included in your re-evaluation will depend on your individual status. If your body is fragile and your pain is easily aggravated, then your re-evaluation will not include a full re-test of your measurements. In that case you will be working to keep your pain down long enough to start the exercises in the Corrective Program; a complete re-test could be counterproductive. You might have re-measurements of a few areas to see how things are going, but not at the risk of losing the progress you have fought so hard for. If your body is not as fragile, or once you are feeling better, you should have a re-evaluation of your measurements every 12 weeks until you reach your goals. The re-measurements will reveal whether the exercises are effective or not.

YELLOW: Study Chapter 5, Your Protective Program. In the YELLOW group you start both the Protective Program and the Corrective Program in the first couple of weeks. In the Protective Program, work on Step 1 as much as you can prior to the physical therapy evaluation. Step 2 in this chapter can take from one week to several months depending on your mechanical limitations. You will hopefully achieve Step 3, the Quick-Relief Strategy, in the first week. Your PT should work on all the steps of your Protective Program with you.

Finding the answers for Steps 2 and 3 should be easier for you than for those in the RED group. If you are closer to the RED group, you might spend more time developing and using Steps 2 and 3. If you are closer to the GREEN group, you only have a short period of time to learn about your specific back positions and how they relate to your pain before your pain decreases; once you start pursuing helpful positions and performing the right exercises your pain might quickly subside. The problem with your pain subsiding quickly is that your learning opportunity is gone. Take advantage of the time you have to learn what your pain is telling you, because when your pain is gone your underlying problems still exists. You ultimately have more control if you are aware of the specific back positions and how they influence your pain during activity.

YELLOW: Study Chapter 6, Your Corrective Program. In the YELLOW group you vary significantly in how you develop your Corrective Program, because some of you are closer to the RED group and some of you are closer to the GREEN group.

- *Range of Motion:* The majority of you should have the initial program of range of motion exercises in the first two months.
- *Motor Control:* The majority of you should have the initial motor control activity in the first month. If you are struggling with the first recommended trunk stabilization exercise, make sure you do not start others until you can perform that first exercise for 30 seconds.
- *Strength:* Strengthening can take 1-6 months to start depending on how irritable your back and legs are.
- *Posture:* You can start postural activities once your other mechanics improve, particularly range of motion.

YELLOW: Study Chapter 7, Exercises. You can use this chapter to reinforce your exercise technique for exercises that the PT selects for you. You can use the DVD as well for those specific exercises. When your PT needs to modify any of your exercises listen to your PT's instructions and not the book or DVD instructions.

GREEN GROUP

Description of GREEN:

There are generally two types of scenarios for frequency, intensity and duration in the GREEN group.

In the first scenario the pain can range from 1/10 to 9/10. This pain occurs with a substantial activity such as a high level athletic activity or a prolonged heavy chore. The more intense pain occurs only during the activity and then drops to a lower intensity for a few days before going away. This pain could happen a couple times every year when doing a very heavy activity or sports training routine. This could also happen every week. The weekly pain can go on for several weeks to months. If it goes on for longer than a couple of months, you need to consider looking at the issues for the YELLOW group. The key with the GREEN group is that your daily activities of dressing, bathing, grooming, household chores, social activities, and work are not the activities that increase your pain. They are not affected other than a few days after the activity that aggravated the pain.

In the other scenario the pain occurs during daily activities. In this case the pain is at a very low intensity, 1/10 - 2/10, and results from a repetitive or prolonged activity lasting 5 minutes or so. Or it is a very sharp intense pain above a 5/10 that occurs after a heavy activity and resolves quickly, in a few seconds. Most people in this group are seeking help to prevent their problems from getting worse. They often report that although their pain is not intense or frequent they are pursuing help because they do not want to become like their parents, who were ultimately crippled with pain.

In both cases your daily self-care activities including dressing, bathing, grooming, and light-to-moderate household chores like cooking and cleaning are not disrupted by the pain.

Usually you do not have pain with most heavy household chores, just with the one that causes the pain. Sometimes after the pain is aggravated, you might feel it with other heavy household chores.

Customizing Chapters for GREEN:

GREEN: Study Chapter 3, Back Pain and Basic Human Mechanics.

GREEN: Study Chapter 4, System Limitations Evaluation, and seek out a physical therapist for your evaluation.

- *History:* Provide as detailed, measurable, and objective a description as possible. Work on the first step of the Protective Program and bring your written information to the evaluation. Your PT needs as much information about your pain as possible because your pain will resolve quickly. You will need that information down the road to make the best judgments about what is going on when you have pain during complicated activities.
- *Postural Evaluation:* Most of you can have the entire postural evaluation.
- *Range of Motion Evaluation:* Most of you can have the entire ROM evaluation.
- *Motor Control Evaluation:* The physical therapist can assess your motor control.
- *Strength Evaluation, (Manual Muscle Test or MMT) :* Most of you can have all or part of the manual muscle test. How much of the test depends on your individual back issues and back irritability. If the MMT is not performed in the first session it will be performed when you can tolerate it, which for most of you is within 8 weeks.
- *Re-evaluation:* The re-measurements are very important. The GREEN group should be able to tolerate re-measurements for ROM 12 weeks after the program is in full swing and for strength 12 weeks after the strength exercise program is in full swing. You should have re-measurements until you reach your goals. The re-measurements will reveal whether the exercises are effective or not.

GREEN: Study Chapter 5, Your Protective Program. In this chapter work on as much of the first step as you can prior to your physical therapy evaluation. Your PT will work on all the steps with you. You will need to concentrate on the second step right away. Your opportunity for learning will be very short, because your pain will probably decrease quickly. The pain gives you important information to help you understand what is going on for your back. If you know about the nature of your pain, you will be more able to figure out what part of the complicated activity is causing the pain. This will be more difficult for you than for REDS and YELLOWS because you do not have immediate or regular feedback from your pain. You will hopefully achieve step 3, the Quick-Relief Strategy, in the first week.

GREEN: Study Chapter 6, Your Corrective Program. Concentrate on all four areas. Within 6-10 sessions you should have your initial exercise program, which includes stretching, motor control and strengthening. Your initial Corrective Program should address all major limitations in range of motion and strength, and it should include trunk stabilization exercises to improve motor control. Your postural activities will be added at the re-evaluation when you demonstrate improvement in your mechanics. The 12-week measurements are very important to assure an effective program.

Your Corrective Program should be easier to develop than for either of the other groups because you have fewer limitations and less pain to take into consideration.

- *Range of Motion:* You should have your initial program developed in 6-10 sessions.
- *Motor Control:* You should have motor control exercises within the first 6-10 sessions. If you are struggling with the first recommended trunk stabilization exercise, make sure you do not start others until you can perform that exercise for 30 seconds.
- *Strength:* You should have your first full strengthening program within the first two months, depending on how often you attend physical therapy.
- *Posture:* You will start postural activities once your mechanics improve and allow you to safely work on improved posture.

GREEN: Study Chapter 7, Exercises. You can use this chapter to reinforce your technique for exercises that the PT selects for you. You can use the DVD as well for those specific exercises. When your PT needs to modify any of your exercises listen to your PT's instructions and not the book or DVD instructions.

CAUTION:

A caution for those of you who think you are in the GREEN or YELLOW group. If you have significant discomfort after the evaluation or when you begin the treatment programs, you might be more closely related to the group that is more involved. You might be a very well-controlled YELLOW instead of a GREEN, or a very-controlled RED instead of a YELLOW. Some of you have, consciously or unconsciously, altered your activities to avoid pain, and so your level of pain can be deceiving. Underneath there could be more problems than you realize. In this case following the recommendations for a group that is less involved and more rapidly progressing through the program might result in increased pain, revealing a greater depth of underlying problems. In this case you need to follow the recommendations for the next more involved group. You might also be more involved than you thought you were if you have been taking medication to decrease your pain.

CHAPTER 3

Back Pain And Basic Human Mechanics

WHAT IS PAIN?

IN my opinion, your pain is not the real problem. It is your body's warning system to alert your brain that you have a problem.

If you break your leg and do not feel pain, you might just keep using your leg and further damage it. Pain informs you if you have a stomach ulcer, a tumor, or a tooth cavity, or if you are in the midst of having a heart attack. In all of these cases no one suggests that you try to just make the pain go away and let the real underlying problem persist. To me it does not make sense to simply eliminate or mask the pain from the back either. It is important to listen to what the pain is trying to tell you and to learn what you can about your underlying problems. Pain can be a wise teacher that, if listened to, can help you immensely.

In this System Limitations Approach, pain serves as a source of information. It works as an Alarm, a Guard, a Mentor for Positions, a Guide during Treatment, and a Consultant about your Progress. It is essential that you to grasp the idea that pain has different roles to play in the identification of your underlying problem and during the development of your treatment programs. You can refer back to this section when you are working to develop your programs and are better at listening to your pain.

Pain is not something to be afraid of. Many people become frightened by their pain and think it means they need to go to bed and/or stop activity. Use the many roles of pain to help you learn about your body, your pain and the most helpful activities for you.

Pain is also a source of motivation. People are generally interested in working on their back problems as long as they have pain. I have found with a number of patients that when the pain is gone so is the program. But when the pain initially goes away the underlying problems still exist, so if you stop your program your pain generally returns. If this happens to you, ask yourself if you performed the program long enough to address your underlying problems. If not, did you at least resume the program that decreased your pain? Better yet, make a promise to yourself to stay with your program after the pain is gone and continue until you find you have done as much as you can to address your underlying problems. Then develop a plan to maintain that progress.

THE MANY ROLES OF PAIN

ALARM

Pain is a warning sign that you have a problem. The pattern for many people is that in the beginning the pain provides a little warning, if not listened to it gets stronger and more frequent. For some this takes place over months; for others it occurs over years or decades. Eliminating the pain and not addressing the underlying problem is like turning off the fire alarm and ignoring the burning house. Or like driving down the road with a flat tire and not fixing it. When you keep driving on the flat tire you run the risk of further damaging the car. Similarly, for back pain, I believe that eliminating the pain and not addressing the underlying problems can result in more wear and tear on the spine.

GUARD

While the pain is present, it guards you from activities that require mechanical abilities you don't have, given your mechanical limitations. As a guard the pain might prevent you from doing certain activities, or at least make you think twice before engaging in those activities. When the pain is gone, so is the guard. When you first feel pain-free and your guard is gone, you might pursue an activity you were unable to do just days before, only to end up in significant pain. This is because, at some level, the underlying problem still exists. I often tell people that they will have their greatest pain after they are their most pain-free, since there is no guard to caution them about their activity and they pursue activities that exceed their abilities.

So while your pain is present, learn what it is telling you about what your back can and cannot tolerate. When your pain is gone, your new pain-inspired insight becomes your guard.

The tricky part about relying on your insight as your guard is knowing what previously painful activities you can start to do as you make progress. Working with a physical therapist who helps you methodically resume your activities will help you with this challenge.

MENTOR FOR POSITIONS

Your pain can be a great mentor, helping you learn about specific back positions that increase or decrease your pain. Your PT will have you move your back through the following positions: arched, flattened, side bend right, side bend left, rotate right and rotate left. You will note which of the specific positions of your back increase your pain, which decrease your pain, and which result in no change in pain. Then you use that information to learn how to position your back during activity.

Learning which specific back positions increase and decrease your pain is a significant part of building your Protective Program. Armed with that information, you learn to go through your day avoiding those specific back positions that increase your pain and to pursue those specific back positions that decrease your pain.

One painful movement to highlight is when the pain indicates that some tissue inside is getting pinched. Be aware of pain that increases on the side of the joint that is moving together. The best example to illustrate this is when you bend your trunk to the right side and the pain increases on the right side; see Figure 3-1a and Figure 3-1b.

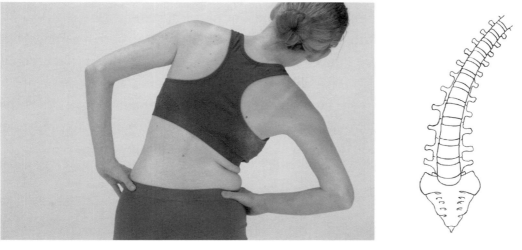

Fig. 3-1a   *Fig. 3-1b*

When that happens learn to modify or avoid activities that require your back to lean to the right, to protect whatever tissue is being aggravated. As your overall mechanics improve, you might note that you no longer have pain when you bend to the right.

GUIDE DURING TREATMENT

The original pain and new pains can guide your treatment. If the original pain increases as a result of an exercise, you learn that that particular exercise is not helpful at this time. If the original pain decreases, you learn that the exercise is helpful. In this way the pain helps guide the development of your exercise program. I do not believe in "no pain no gain." We want to build an exercise program that addresses your limitations and does not increase your pain.

Because the Corrective Program focuses specifically on the limitations that cause the back pain, you are at risk of aggravating your pain. A slight change in the exercise technique can result in the movement that causes your pain. Hopefully your pain will let you know that there is a problem with the technique before you do it long enough to really aggravate the problem. You can then make any needed adjustments to the exercise. The Corrective Program should not increase the original back pain. However, other pains might pop up; following are suggestions of how to manage those pains.

During treatment you will start to have new pains. Despite your back pain, parts of your body are actually happy in their present physical state. Like the employees who are not doing their jobs in the example in Chapter 1, some parts of your body have been on vacation and are not interested in coming back to work. So when you start working to improve your mechanics, those areas speak up with all sorts of new sensations. Report all of these new sensations to your PT. You will not address most of them, because most of these issues resolve themselves; if you start chasing all of the new sensations your forward progress slows down.

In some instances the new pain is a sign that your present physical state is a way to steer clear of an old problem, and your present effort to correct and shift back might cause that old problem to rear its ugly head. On a couple of occasions I have had to tell patients that I thought that correcting their present problems might possibly bring on a whole new set of problems, and they needed to decide whether they wanted to risk that or keep the problems they currently had. In those cases the people went on to address their problems and managed fine. Although rare, perhaps your present problems are your best case scenario. Your PT will help you with this sorting-out process.

Some new pains that need to be addressed are:

- red flags indicating a potential serious problem
- yellow flags indicating problems
- new pains or sensations that are not resolving themselves
- new pains that concern you but do not fall into either category
- new pains that your PT feels might generate other problems

CONSULTANT ABOUT PROGRESS

While the Guide During Treatment is about your response to each individual exercise, the Consultant about Progress is about your response to the overall program.

Pain gives you feedback about the progress of both your Protective Program and your Corrective Program. If you have an effective Protective Program and are following it, the feedback is a decrease in the original pain. If you are following an effective Corrective Program, you are making progress with your body's underlying problems and the feedback is a consistent ability to perform previously painful activities.

While you track your progress it's important to keep in mind the following two exceptions.

1) The absence of pain does not necessarily mean you have made progress.

You could have less pain merely by chance. In this case you did not actively do anything to decrease your pain; you did not learn anything, but simply by chance you avoided those activities that increase your pain and thus the absence of pain is really luck, not a sign of progress.

2) The presence of pain does not necessarily mean you have lost progress.

An intermittent increase in pain can signal that you performed an activity beyond your current mechanical abilities. This is not a sign that you have lost ground or had a setback. It simply warns that you are not ready for that activity yet. If you *repeatedly* do activities that ask too much of your back, you could have a setback and your back could get worse.

ANATOMY

For the System Limitations Approach to Pain, you need a general idea of what is going on inside your body. It is important for you to be familiar with the following:

- JOINTS: You move only at your joints. You need to know where your joints are. When you move your body, think about which joint the motion comes from to move you into the different position.
- BONES: Bones provide structure and bear weight. They also serve as a place for your muscles to attach.
- SOFT TISSUE: For our purposes, soft tissue is everything other than bones. Soft tissue includes the muscles (contracting to move your body), tendons (attaching muscles to bones), ligaments (attaching bones to bones), nerves (transmitting information between the brain and the body), and the joint capsules (balloon-like structures that surround many joints). I often say to patients that if it were not for soft tissue we would be a pile of bones on the floor. It appears that the condition of your soft tissue is what sets up the relationship of your bones. If the tissue on one side of a joint is short and lacks flexibility while the tissue on the other side is overstretched, then the joint will be subjected to uneven forces. I believe the soft tissue drives the position of the joint in many cases.
- ALIGNMENT: How you line up is important to the health of your body parts. If your body is out of alignment, it causes stress and wear and tear on your structures. In my opinion, your soft tissue has considerable influence on your alignment.

Figure 3-2a presents the anatomical names used in this book and demonstrates the bone structure, joints, and ideal alignment. In Figure 3-2b note the size of the joints. The shoulders and the hips are large ball joints and the joints in the spine are much smaller joints. Which joints look better designed to move you? The shoulder and hip joints are designed for a good deal of motion. The joints in the spine are designed for far less motion.

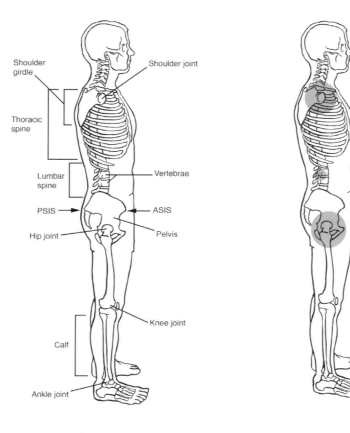

Fig. 3-2a   Fig. 3-2b

THE NEUTRAL SPINE

The position of your spine is important for the health of your back. Dr. Christophe Boulay and his colleagues have researched human alignment, specifically looking at the human body from a side view. [11] What I like about their research is how it seems to fit well with what I see in practice. First, in more scientific terms, they discuss that if your spine is not well balanced, for instance the lower spine is too arched or too flat and your body cannot compensate well for that, then there is a greater opportunity for problems. Secondly they relate the position of the spine to the principle of economy.

The research states, "If for a patient, the measured lordosis is out of the confidence limits of the predicted lordosis, the standing posture is no longer in the conditions of the principle of economy."[12] Followed by, "Ways of adaptation between the spine and pelvis are unbalanced and can improve pathological patterns on a long or short-term basis." [13]

There are forces on your back every day; forces from gravity and from muscle activity. You want to minimize how much these forces impact your spine in a destructive way. You want to pursue a position that is economical, a position that will deal well with the forces on your spine to keep your spine as healthy as possible.

Neutral spine is the term that is commonly used to describe the position that is thought to deal best with the forces on your spine. The generally accepted definition for the position of the neutral spine, from the side is, a slight arch in the lower spine with a level pelvis: meaning the point on the front (ASIS) and the point on the back (PSIS) are level with each other; see Figure 3-3a. However, just like our faces look different, our boney structures are slightly different and therefore the neutral position, or the position that best deals with the forces on the back, will also be slightly different for everyone.

You want your back to *be able to* move into positions other than the neutral position. However, you don't want your back *forced* into another position. Being out of the economical position leads to positions that can become more pathological, meaning more wear and tear on your body; see Figure 3-3b.

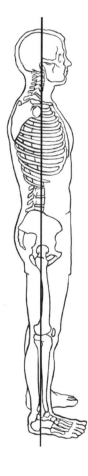
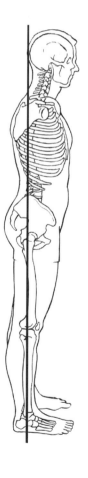

Fig. 3-3a   *Fig. 3-3b*

From the back the neutral spine is positioned vertically straight up from the pelvis; see Figure 3-4a. There are shifts in posture that can be seen from the back and I believe that research will find that they too are less economical, leading to forces on the spine that can cause wear and tear; for example, see Figure 3-4b.

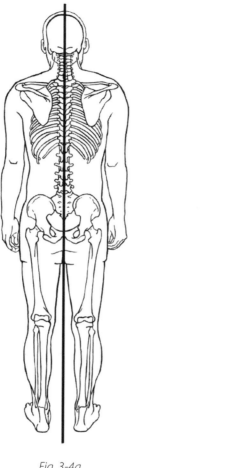

Fig. 3-4a   *Fig. 3-4b*

Each individual bone in the spine is called a vertebra. Each vertebra has a large circular part called the vertebral body. The vertebral body is designed to bear the weight of our body. The joints are located in the back part of the vertebra. The joints are where the vertebra contact and allow motion between the vertebral bones; see Figure 3-5.

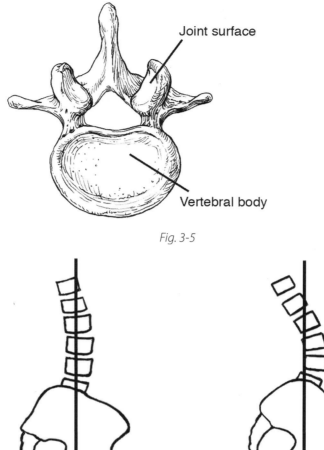

Joint surface

Vertebral body

Fig. 3-5

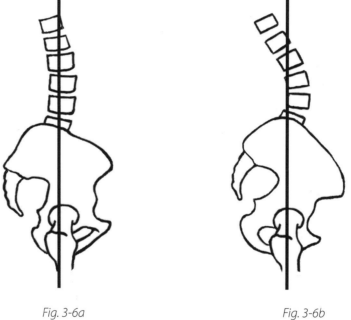

Fig. 3-6a   *Fig. 3-6b*

In the neutral spine position your spine is aligned so that most of your body weight is supported down through the vertebral bodies and not through the joints in the back; see Figure 3-6a. When your spine is out of neutral for example, the arch in your back is increased, the forces are changed, and can cause degenerative changes in the spine; see Figure 3-6b.

In this approach you work to improve your spine's position by addressing the mechanical limitations that affect the position of the spine.

THE BIG FOUR MECHANICS OF HUMAN MOVEMENT

Humans have *mechanics* in order to move, just as mechanics enable an automobile to run. The major *mechanics* that humans need to move are 1) range of motion, 2) strength, 3) motor control, and 4) postural alignment. I call these The Big Four Mechanics. Humans have other tools that contribute to movement, such as sensation and joint play. These will be looked at more specifically as needed on an individual basis. The Big Four Mechanics form the base of the System Limitations Evaluation.

THE BIG FOUR MECHANICS:

1. RANGE OF MOTION

2. STRENGTH

3. MOTOR CONTROL

4. POSTURAL ALIGNMENT

The Big Four Mechanics are needed to perform activity while achieving and maintaining a neutral spine. This includes activities such as sitting, standing, lying down, and walking. The following elaborates on these four mechanics and their important role in maintaining a healthy back.

1. RANGE OF MOTION

The only way you move is through motion at your joints. Range of motion (ROM) stands for the specific distance through which each joint moves. Each activity requires a certain range of motion from each joint in order to perform the activity in a manner that is healthy for your body.

The shoulder and hip joints are ball-and-socket joints designed for considerable motion in six different directions. The knees are large joints, but move in just two directions.

Since your knee joints only bend and straighten, note that when you perform big body movements the only joints to provide rotation and bending to the side are the hip joints and the spine. If you are limited in the hip joints the movement will come from your spine.

The spine is made up of very small joints that are not designed for a great deal of motion. The upper two thirds of the back is attached to a rib cage, significantly limiting motion in that area of the spine; therefore motion in the spine primarily comes from the lower five joints known as the lumbar spine.

2. STRENGTH

While range of motion provides a place from which to move, strength is the muscle power that actually moves your body. The following are properties to be aware of while learning about your mechanics and developing an effective treatment program to improve your mechanics:

- Each muscle has a primary movement that it performs and other movements that it is designed to assist with.
- Some muscles are power muscles that contract very powerfully for a short period of time. An example is your biceps muscle in the front of your upper arm. It produces a lot of power to pick up something heavy, but will not easily tolerate having to hold something heavy for a long period of time; for instance while you wait for someone to open a door.
- Some muscles are postural muscles that contract at a low level for a long period of time. An example would be the muscles along your spine that hold you up for hours while you work at the computer.
- You want to train a muscle in the manner in which it functions. In this case power muscles need exercise with heavier weight held for a shorter period of time, and postural muscles need exercise with lighter weight held for a longer period of time.

3. MOTOR CONTROL

Motor control is the tool your brain uses to coordinate your body's activity, controlling what part of your body moves and what stays still. Dr. Shirley Stockmeyer, a former teacher of mine, defined four stages of motor control; mobility, stability, controlled mobility and skill. Although many aspects of motor control are important for your back what I believe you should focus on is the ability to control your back position while you are active and at rest.

Ideally for your back the trunk is the stable base from which your shoulders move your arms to manipulate your environment and from which your hips move your legs to get you around the environment.

For appropriate motor control you need to have the range of motion and strength in your trunk, arms, and legs that is required for the specific activity you are performing, so that you do not have compensatory activity causing you to perform the activity with faulty motor control.

4. POSTURE

In this System Limitations Approach to Pain, posture is not about whether you are slouching and then correcting to a better position. Repetitive posture, good posture, and poor posture influence your body and will be addressed in the Protective Program. However in this section the focus on posture is about your ability to achieve ideal alignment in standing.

Ideal standing posture is standing straight with your ears over your shoulders, shoulders over hip joints, and hip joints over knees and ankles while your spine has the appropriate curves. I think considering ideal posture as the most economical is an important way to view posture; you want to move as close as you can to ideal posture so that the forces on your spine are the least costly to your spine. For example when your spine moves away from the most economical posture to a more arched or more flattened position, the forces on your spine can be more costly and increase the opportunity for problems.

THE BIG FOUR MECHANICAL LIMITATIONS AND BACK PAIN

The mechanical limitations initially explored in the System Limitations Approach to Pain are 1) decreased range of motion, 2) decreased strength, 3) poor motor control (poor trunk stabilization), and 4) poor postural alignment. These are The Big Four Mechanical Limitations. The main subject of this book is how limitations in the body affect the back. When you have limitations, one of two things primarily occurs: 1) Your back is forced to compensate for limited motion or strength elsewhere in your body, and/or 2) Your back suffers the consequences of poor positioning because of mechanical limitations.

In the first instance the back does its own job *and* the job of another part of the body. This places extra force and activity on the back. The back does more work than it was originally designed to do; eventually it hurts and in some cases experiences wear and tear on the spine.

In the second instance the back can be repeatedly put into a poor position, leading to wear and tear on the spine.

This section discusses each of the limitations more specifically so that you'll have some foundation upon which to understand your own limitations. There are as many combinations of mechanical limitations and pain as there are people who have back pain. Your PT will help make the connections between your limitations and your pain.

The Big Four Mechanical Limitations

1. DECREASED RANGE OF MOTION

2. DECREASED STRENGTH

3. POOR MOTOR CONTROL

4. POOR POSTURAL ALIGNMENT

---

1. DECREASED RANGE OF MOTION

The problem begins for your back when you have limitations in motion that you need for an activity and you still perform that activity, such as, sitting, standing, walking, or running. Now when you sit, stand, walk, or run the motion has to come from another joint. In the case of back pain, the joints in the back are usually where the substitute motion comes from. There are several examples of this in the section entitled, The Impact of Mechanical Limitations on the Back.

A key finding that demonstrates a relationship between your pain and your mechanical limitations is:

> Your back compensates for the limitations in your range of motion; and the position your back uses to compensate for the limitations is one of the specific back positions that increases your pain (See Chapter 5, Step 2a).

In the System Limitations Approach to Pain, the PT: 1) evaluates your range of motion and identifies limitations that force your back to compensate, 2) determines if the position your back uses to compensate for your limited range of motion is a specific back position that increases your pain, 3) determines if the specific back position that increases your pain is the same position your back uses during activities that increase your pain, and 4) designs exercises to address the ROM with your back in the neutral or most pain-free position. Improving range of motion appears to be the greatest factor in decreasing pain.

2. DECREASED STRENGTH

Improving strength appears to be the greatest factor in helping to consistently perform activities with decreased pain. Decreased strength can result in two big problems: 1) The loss of strength in one area forces another area to substitute the strength required to perform an activity. With back pain, it is typically the back that compensates for loss of strength in other areas. 2) The trunk is not strong enough to hold the back in its neutral position during activity. Note the following are examples:

- If you move to stand up and you do not have enough strength in your leg muscles to push you up to standing, even if you try to use your legs for good body mechanics you will recruit the muscles in your back to help you get into an upright position. The muscles in your back were not designed to be responsible for this movement.
- If you do not have adequate strength in your shoulder muscles and you try to push or pull something heavier than your arm muscles can manage alone, you will ask the muscles in your lower back to help.
- During exercises, many people use more weight than the muscles they are trying to strengthen can handle alone. Therefore they recruit strength from other parts of their body, such as the back, to help perform the exercises.
- When there is not enough strength in the trunk, it is difficult to control and protect the neutral spine position.

Your physical therapist identifies your strength limitations with a manual muscle test, and then plans an exercise program to address your limitations. Do not assume you have proper strength. I evaluated a woman who had back pain and the manual muscle test for strength revealed that most of the muscles in one leg were not strong enough to lift the leg itself. If the muscles were not strong enough to lift the weight of the leg, they were not strong enough to carry the weight of the body during standing, walking and many other activities; her back had to do considerable compensating during those activities.

It is important to train muscles for the job they are designed to do. If you want to be a strong swimmer, you don't train for swimming by downhill skiing or skydiving. To improve the function of your body as a unified mechanical system, it is important to strengthen your muscles for the job they are designed to do. You will understand better how to accomplish this as you read Chapters 6 and 7.

3. POOR MOTOR CONTROL

The two parts of poor motor control that are important in back pain are: 1) the inability to move your back into the neutral position, or 2) the inability to keep your back in a neutral position during activity.

Your goal is to train your body to position and protect your back in the neutral position during activity, without having to consciously think about it. We want your back to be able to move in and out of the neutral position we just don't want it to have to be forced out of the neutral position, or for you to not have the control and coordination to support the back in the neutral position during activity.

To develop motor control for the back you should focus on trunk stabilization exercises. A repetitive activity using the arms and the legs for movement while controlling the back position.

To keep your back stable during trunk stabilization exercises you need to have the range of motion and strength in your arms and legs that is required to perform the activity.

4. POOR POSTURAL ALIGNMENT

In the System Limitations Approach to Pain your PT will evaluate your best upright posture and compare it to the ideal upright posture for humans. The limitations in your best alignment reflect limitations in the other three mechanics: range of motion, strength, and motor control.

Poor alignment also suggests that you are not in an economical position. You are in a position that is more costly and more harmful. The everyday forces on your back are not distributed ideally and can lead to wear and tear on your spine. It is okay to move in and out of other postures and positions, but you don't want to be forced to assume and maintain poor positions.

In this approach your alignment is considered to be a reflection of limitations in your other mechanics. It is strongly recommended that you do not try to improve your posture until you start to improve the other three mechanics. If you try to force better alignment, not only will you have difficulty achieving the alignment but you can unknowingly place more stress on your body's structures, possibly causing increased pain.

The key in the long run to functioning with a better, more economical posture, lies in your ability to improve all of your mechanics and then work to achieve your best postural alignment.

THE IMPACT OF MECHANICAL LIMITATIONS ON THE BACK

When you find that you have mechanical limitations, the next step is for your PT to see if the limitations relate to the positions of your back that increase your pain. It is easy to illustrate in a book the effect of decreased range of motion on the back. It is quite difficult in a book to illustrate the effect of decreased strength and poor motor control. Following are examples of how limitations in range of motion impact the position of the back during activity.

The following examples focus on the effect of one limitation on the back. The line from A to B represents the area of range of motion that we are focusing on. The first illustration demonstrates normal range of motion; the hip is in the position designed for the activity and the back is in the neutral position. The second illustration represents a limitation in the hip range of motion and the effect on the body position when the back does not compensate for the limitation. The third illustration represents the limitation in hip range of motion and reveals what happens when the back compensates for the limited range of motion.

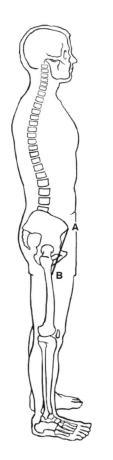

Fig. 3-7a
Full hip extension

Back in neutral

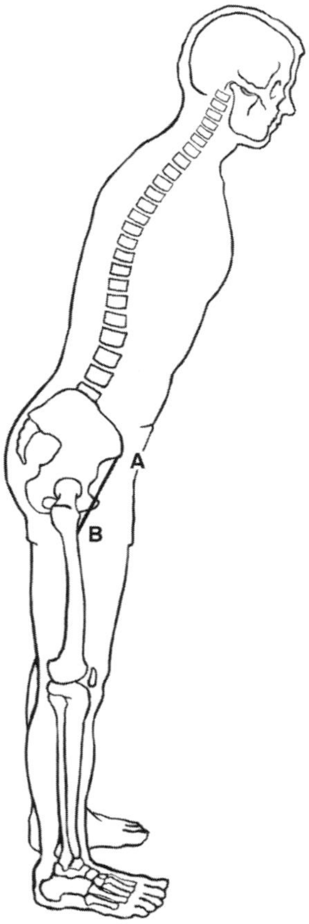

Fig. 3-7b
Limited hip extension

Back does not compensate

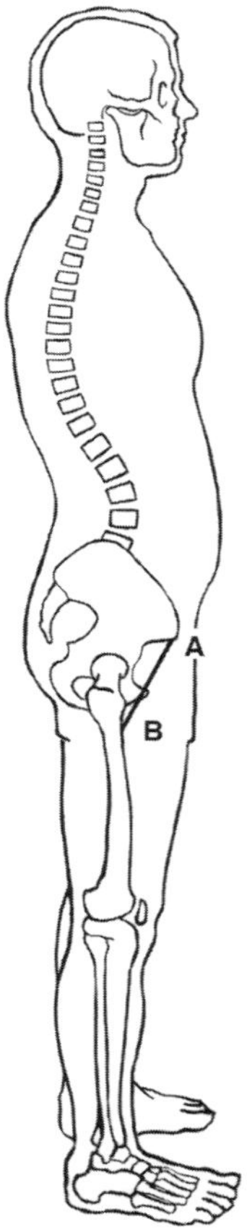

Fig. 3-7c
Limited hip extension

Back compensates

For standing you need full hip extension to have your legs under your body and let your back be in neutral above your legs. The line from A to B represents the area where range of motion is needed to let the hip move into extension. The first illustration demonstrates enough hip extension range of motion to let the leg move under your body while your back stays in the neutral position; see Figure 3-7a. The line from A to B in the next two illustrations represents decreased range of motion that does not allow full hip extension. In this case you have to either lean forward to keep your back in neutral; see Figure 3-7b, or you have to arch your back to compensate for the limited hip extension range of motion; see Figure 3-7c.

If you do not have full hip extension range of motion, the limitation can cause your back to arch every time you stand. This can lead to compression in the joints in the spine, which can lead to degenerative changes in the joints. If that happens whenever you are standing imagine how the force on your spine could wear your back down and become painful.

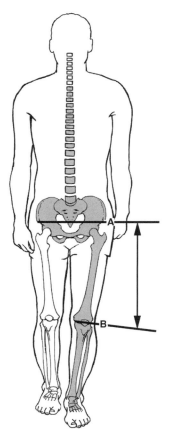 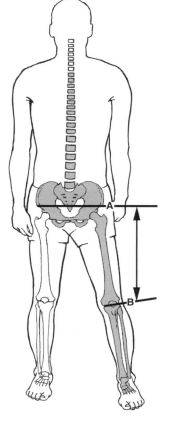 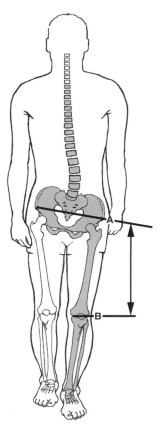

Fig. 3-8a

Full hip adduction

Back in neutral

Fig. 3-8b

Limited hip adduction

Back does not compensate

Fig. 3-8c

Limited hip adduction

Back compensates

Walking requires one leg to move under your body to support you as your other leg swings forward. Hip adduction is the motion you use at your hip joint to move your leg under your body. The line from A to B, in this example, represents the length of the tissue on the outside of the hip and thigh. A limitation in the length of this tissue can limit hip adduction and thereby limit the hip joints ability to move the leg underneath you.

The first illustration demonstrates enough hip adduction range of motion and length in the tissue on the outside of the thigh to let the leg move underneath you while the back stays in the neutral position; see Figure 3-8a. The line from A to B in the next two illustrations represents decreased range of motion, and so there is not enough range of motion to let the hip joint move your leg underneath you. In this case your leg has to stay out to the side in order to keep your hips level and your back in neutral, as seen in Figure 3-8b; or you move your leg underneath you which causes your hip to drop down and your back to bend sideways, as seen in Figure 3-8c. In other words, your back bends sideways to compensate for the lack of hip motion and provide the motion to move your leg underneath you

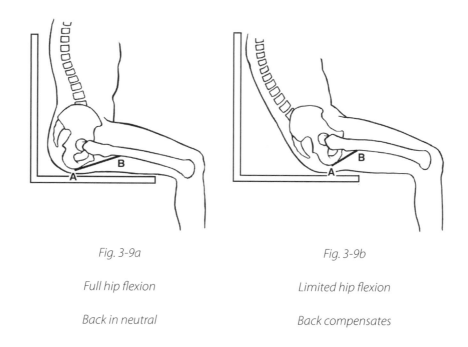

Fig. 3-9a

Full hip flexion

Back in neutral

Fig. 3-9b

Limited hip flexion

Back compensates

In most cases when you want to sit you need to bend 90 degrees at your hip joints, as there is a 90 degree angle between the seat and the back of the chair. The line from A to B represents the area where range of motion is needed to let you bend 90 degrees at the hip. The first illustration demonstrates enough range of motion for the hip to bend while the back stays in the neutral position; see Figure 3-9a. In the second illustration there is limited range of motion represented by the shortened line from A to B, in this case the back has to flatten to compensate for the lack of hip motion and to achieve the bend needed between the trunk and the legs; see Figure 3-9b. In this case because of the back of the chair the back does not have the option to stay in neutral with this type of limitation.

The only way to compensate for a lack of hip motion and maintain the back in neutral while sitting is to sit in a chair where the back of the seat reclines and less of a bend is required at the hip.

There are more involved compensations for limitations. People usually have multiple limitations occurring simultaneously that contribute to back pain. I have never had a case in which someone complained of pain and had only one limitation. My sense is that the back and the body tolerate compensating for one limitation. Some patterns of limitations are quite involved.

WHAT'S HAPPENING IN YOUR BACK?

Following are some of the possibilities I believe could be taking place in your back. This is a great area for research.

- There are no signs of wear and tear in your back. Your back pain is the result of your back doing too much by compensating for decreased range of motion or strength in another part of your body. Some joints in your spine could be moving more than they are designed to move, yet no changes show up on the X-ray or MRI of your spine.
- There are no signs of wear and tear in your back. Your back pain results from your back being repeatedly poorly positioned, due to limitations in trunk strength and/or stability. You could have constant compression in the joints of your spine leading to degeneration in the joints, yet this is not shown in an X-ray or MRI of your spine.
- There are signs of wear and tear in your back, minimal to significant changes such as, degenerative changes in the joints of your spine, herniated discs, poor alignment, and possibly too much movement seen in the joints in your spine. These changes could be a result of your back doing too much by compensating for decreased range of motion or strength in another part of your body, or they could result from being poorly positioned repeatedly due to limitations in trunk strength and/or stability. This scenario appears to be more common in those with a long history of pain and who present with significant limitations in range of motion.

CAUSES

The first question most people ask during their evaluation after they have seen and felt the limitations in their mechanics is, "How did this happen?" You might never get a specific answer. I believe that for most of us a combination of factors makes us uniquely *us* in our physical limitations:

- ANATOMICAL HEREDITY: Our bodies are all structured to perform the same tasks. For example, we all have hearts and lungs that we use in the same way for the same reason. However, other than identical twins no two people have the same structure, the same face with the same cheek bones, or the same structure elsewhere in our bodies. You have inherited your structures, and they are different from the structures of your neighbors, co-workers, etc., and so you have different strengths and weaknesses and these can lead to different problems in mechanics.
- FAMILY TENDENCIES: If a father walks with a spring in his step, most likely you will see that in the children as well, they copy their parents' ways of moving. A change in a pattern of movement such as walking can have an influence on your mechanics, for better or worse.
- CHILDHOOD AND ADULT ACTIVITIES: Repetitive activities such as occupational or sports activities influence your body. You can see the effect of swimming and gymnastics on the development of young bodies.
- ACCIDENTS AND INJURIES: Changes in the mechanics in your body after a big accident or a small injury can change the way you move. After an accident or injury it is important to work to regain all of the mechanics that you can in range of motion, strength, trunk stabilization, and posture.

- OUR CULTURE: I believe cultural issues play a role in mechanical pain. In many cultures we sit in a chair for a tremendous amount of time, from 5 years old to 18 years old in school, in the car, at the computer, for dinner, watching TV, etc., and then one day we wonder why we can't sit without pain or why we have pain when we move from sitting to standing. I have also noticed that cultural patterns appear to affect mechanics. For example, in Hawaii, flip-flops can be worn year-round and I found significantly fewer limitations in ankle motion. On the mainland, much more time is spent in shoes with heels. Shoes with heels keep the calf muscle in a shortened position. Loss of calf muscle flexibility limits ankle joint motion.

After you add up all your individual factors—your heredity, your family tendencies, your repetitive activities, your accidents and injuries, and your cultural influences—you become uniquely you in your mechanics.

SUMMARY OF MECHANICS

Quite simply, for each activity you need certain mechanics. In some cases of back pain the back is compensating for limitations and in other cases the back pain is a consequence of poor positioning. Each person is an individual, and your pain alerts you to your own unique set of Big Four Mechanical Limitations.

Understanding what is happening in your body requires knowledge of the basics of how the human body moves and how limitations affect that movement. This chapter is designed to help you understand basic body mechanics and pain. Please do not get overwhelmed by the information. You needn't understand everything; you need only understand what applies to *your* limitations and *your* back pain. Know that even though you might have a very good idea of what is going on with your body, you might not find a direct solution to *every* mechanical limitation or *every* pain.

This book cannot discuss everyone's potential issues. Where your pain is located, your back, hips, legs, foot, shoulders, neck, depends on a number of factors: your mechanical limitations, what activities you do, and how you compensate for those limitations. You and your neighbor could have the same limitations but different pain. You perform different activities and compensate differently than your neighbor. Therefore the area that becomes overused or irritated is different for each of you. If you both had limited motion in the hips, one of you could have knee pain while the other could have back pain. Each of you is unique in what is happening to your body and causing your pain.

CHAPTER 4

The System Limitation Evaluation For Back Pain

INTRODUCTION

TO use the System Limitations Approach to Pain for the treatment of back pain, you and your PT start with the System Limitations Evaluation for Back Pain. In my opinion, the measurements recommended for this evaluation are the minimum needed to understand your back pain and your mechanics. However, depending on your problems your PT might not take all of the measurements in the initial evaluation; some measurements might need to wait until you can better tolerate the testing. On the other hand, your PT might include additional measurements as needed.

The intention of this chapter is to add to your understanding of this approach and to help you make an informed judgment as you compare the evaluation you received with the evaluation recommended in this approach.

The tools of this evaluation are the basic tools physical therapists learn in school, taken a few steps further to explore the relationship between your mechanical limitations and your back pain in a measurable way. The parts of the evaluation are:

- A detailed history of your pain is taken to achieve an objective, measurable description of your pain.
- Measurements of your mechanics are taken with attention to the technique to increase the accuracy of the results and to note the impact of the limitations on your neutral spine position.
- The measurements of your mechanics are expanded, measuring joints throughout your body instead of only the region of the pain with merely a cursory look at the rest of your body.
- The PT makes an assessment of your findings to determine whether you have mechanical limitations related to your back pain.
- The treatment program is tailored to you, developed from your limitations, your pain, and your activities.

- Periodic re-evaluations are deemed essential to keep your program on track and to keep you on track.
- Further evaluation of specific issues in your back or in your entire system will be provided, depending on your presentation.

Elements of the System Limitations Evaluation:

1. **History**

   - **Objective, measurable details of your experience with pain and activity**

   - **Your medical history**

2. **Measurements**

   - **Postural alignment**

   - **Range of motion**

   - **Motor control**

   - **Strength**

   - **Additional measurements**

3. **Assessment**

   - **PT's professional opinion of whether you have mechanical limitations that are related to your pain**

4. **Plan**

   - **Your Protective Program**

   - **Your Corrective Program**

   - **Your additional treatment**

5. **Re-Evaluations**

If your PT determines that your pain is inconsistent with your limitations, you need to follow up with your physician to consider other causes of your pain. Of the 15 percent of back pain that is diagnosed most are medical issues such as fractures and tumors. One of the great aspects of this approach is that you relate measurable findings to measurable findings. If you have a fracture, your measurable findings will most likely not be consistent with your pain.

If you have pain that is only partly related to your mechanical limitations, the System Limitations Approach to Pain can be used in combination with other physical therapy treatments and other medical treatments, presuming there are no medical reasons to the contrary.

FINDING A PHYSICAL THERAPIST (PT)

WHAT TO LOOK FOR

First and most importantly, look for a licensed physical therapist to work with you on this *complete* program. Although other practitioners might think they can offer all or parts of this approach, in my experience, physical therapists are uniquely qualified to provide this program. Note: In many countries the professional title is "physiotherapist."

To find out if this approach can help you with your back pain, you need a physical therapist who makes a commitment to both the perspective and the details recommended in this approach, someone who has the support of his or her office or clinic. This is not a cookie-cutter program where one size fits all; rather, you become a project for your PT. You need a sense that your PT is trying to put together the whole picture of what is happening in your body.

How do you find the right physical therapist for you? When seeking a physical therapist who offers this approach, check the website in this book for a list of physical therapists who have indicated an interest in learning about this approach. Being on this list is neither a guarantee of the quality of one's work nor an endorsement. I do not evaluate facilities or therapists, but the list serves as an avenue to help you start looking.

You need a PT you think will work well with you and who will learn what is needed to help you. You might need to shop around to find the right person. The key is to ask pointed questions and pay close attention to the answers.

QUESTIONS TO ASK A PHYSICAL THERAPIST

1. Are you familiar with the System Limitations Approach to Pain and the System Limitations Evaluation?
2. If so, how familiar are you? Have you read this book? Have you been to a talk or seen the DVD for PTs? Have you treated people using this approach?
3. If you've used this approach, what did you think? How many patients have you treated this way? In general, does this approach work for you as a PT? For the patient?
4. If unfamiliar with this approach, are you willing to work with me and learn how to follow it?
5. Are you able to schedule adequate time for the evaluation and for sessions to instruct me in my Protective and Corrective Programs?

6. Will you schedule me to come back at 12-week intervals for a re-evaluation of my progress as needed?

7. Would you work with me each time I come, or would I be treated by multiple therapists?

8. If I can use my medical insurance to pay for treatment through you, will my insurance company's policies influence how long an evaluation you will schedule for me? Will it influence the number of appointments? Will it determine whether you will discharge me when I am ready to work on the programs on my own, or whether you schedule me for re-evaluations and follow-up work at 12-week intervals while I continue to work on my own?

EVALUATING THE ANSWERS

There are several things to watch for and avoid. Look for a licensed physical therapist genuinely interested in helping you. The PT might acknowledge limitations in knowledge of the System Limitations Approach to Pain, or have difficulty scheduling the time needed, but, presuming s/he will work to find a way around these obstacles in order to meet your needs, you might be able to forge an effective partnership. If you find someone unfamiliar with the approach but willing to learn about it, s/he can read this book and go to the website to find other relevant materials.

In the System Limitations Approach you spend more time with your PT during your initial evaluation and in your follow-up sessions to develop your exercise program than is historically scheduled for physical therapy. In my practice I schedule three hours for the evaluation; this is what I find necessary to understand the person's mechanical condition. I schedule one-on-one follow-up appointments for 1-1½ hour sessions to develop the Protective and Corrective Programs. Scheduling the time needed in the beginning is extremely important for the program's success.

You want to avoid an office that does the following: seems reluctant to schedule sufficient time for the PT to accomplish the evaluation in one session; indicates that your one-on-one time for the follow-up sessions will be limited; does not enable you to make all of your appointments with the same PT; or tells you that they use only certain parts of the approach.

Sometimes it is difficult to tell what a clinic is like before you start. Some clinics are known as "production factories," concentrating on how many patients they can see in a day. Let's hope they are rare today. Some other individuals or businesses advertise that they offer a program; yet, they do not have the commitment to pursue the program as recommended. With a facility like this, if you do not do well you're faced with the dilemma of trying another approach or trying this approach again with another PT clinic.

DIFFICULT CIRCUMSTANCES

Over the next few years it will be difficult for some clinics to provide this approach. Physical Therapists treat back pain as well as people who have had strokes, amputations, heart attacks, burns, etc. A PT in the rural setting could be taking care of your neighbor with a stroke and your sister with a fractured arm. This PT may have a difficult time finding the resources, energy, and time to learn a new treatment program with a new way of scheduling. In such circumstances, my hat is off to any PT who would make an attempt to do so.

Finances are another difficulty when starting a new program. Some clinics are already stretched to pay their staff and their bills; it can seem too risky to offer a program if they participate with insurance and the company does not agree to reimburse them. The time initially involved in this approach is more than the third party payers are accustomed too.

If your insurance company's policies are restrictive and will not pay a physical therapist for sufficient time for your evaluation, call the insurance company yourself and present your case. Let them know why you believe this is in the best interest of both you and the insurance company. Or offer to pay for the time needed for the evaluation, and see if insurance will help cover the follow-up sessions. This might seem costly; however, it could pay off in the long run if you've had difficulty finding answers about what is happening to your body and causing your pain.

THE SYSTEM LIMITATIONS EVALUATION FOR BACK PAIN

PATIENT'S HISTORY

<u>Your Experience with Pain and Activity:</u> In the first part of the evaluation you should describe your pain and activity level in as detailed, objective, and measurable terms as possible. This is a big part of your responsibility in the effort to identify the cause of your pain. It is not easy to describe pain. Before your evaluation write your answers to Step 1 in your Protective Program Manual in Chapter 5 and take what you have completed in the manual to your evaluation. Your PT also needs to hear your experience in your own words so as to ask follow-up questions and help you describe your pain in objective and measurable terms.

Your PT needs to hear the whole history of your pain; this includes the time of the first episode of back pain, the general trend over the years, how many episodes a year, how long they lasted, any other pain you have had (neck, shoulder, foot, etc.), any injuries you have had, any previous treatment, what worked and what didn't.

Your detailed description helps you and your PT to: understand what is happening to your body, track your progress in measurable terms, identify activities that are helping or hurting your progress, identify problems in your Protective and Corrective Programs, and make adjustments in your program. The detailed description also helps decide how to manage unresolved issues that you have in the end. In addition, your description helps to keep your motivation up, since you can see your progress in measurable terms. Here is an example:

> Lauren came into treatment with pain from her ankles to her shoulders. Initially cleaning a small apartment caused pain that would force her to bed for four days. A year after beginning treatment with this approach, she went on a hike with her daughter up a mountain that included climbing over a number of obstacles. She said that she was very discouraged when her legs ached after the hike. The PT read Lauren the written account of what her experience had been a year earlier. Lauren said that she had forgotten how bad it had been. She was much happier when she realized how much progress she had made, and was impressed that she was able to go on that vigorous hike and suffer only aching legs instead of ending up in bed for days.

Your Medical History: Your physical therapist needs to know your medical history; including surgeries, illnesses, results from any tests you have had, and a list of medications you take. If you have a medical problem such as asthma or a seizure disorder that can occur during a physical therapy session, inform the PT about what happens when you have an episode and how it is best managed. Add any past injuries you forgot to mention when you described your pain.

From your history, your PT decides which back pain group you most closely resemble—RED, YELLOW, or GREEN, and how much of the evaluation s/he thinks you will tolerate. From your history your PT also determines if you have Red Flags requiring that you see your physician, either prior to the evaluation or, depending on the problem, at some time in the near future.

MEASUREMENTS

Postural Alignment: Postural Alignment will be evaluated first. This is not an evaluation of whether you stand with poor posture; rather, your PT evaluates how well you line up when you try to stand in your best upright position.

To evaluate your posture, you will stand in your best upright position next to a plumb line (a string coming down from the ceiling that represents an upright vertical position) to compare to your alignment. Your PT will evaluate your alignment on all four sides—front, both sides, and back—and note your foot, ankle, knee, hip, pelvis, spine, shoulder, shoulder blade, neck, and head positions. S/he will write down, in as measurable terms as possible, the difference between your posture and the ideal postural alignment. For example, the hip joint is three inches in front of the plumb line. This way you have something measurable to refer back to for comparison.

Your PT might ask if you can make certain adjustments toward a position of better alignment, and observe whether you can move closer to ideal posture or not. The postural findings can indicate the limitations that will be found in the other Big Four Mechanics, which is why posture is evaluated first. *Remember that it is too early to try to <u>correct</u> your postural alignment at this time. You probably have some mechanical limitations that limit your ability to achieve the ideal upright position, and improvement in your mechanics needs to come before improvement in your posture.*

<u>Range of Motion:</u> Range of motion (ROM) measurements let you know how much movement you have. Each body motion has an already established range that is considered normal. If you do not have the normal range, you have a limitation in your range of motion. In this approach, the PT pays special attention to whether you have limitations in a motion required for an activity that causes your back pain.

When measuring ROM, the following guidelines are important:

- The technique used for the measurement must ensure that only the joint being measured is moving. Ideally the joint above and below the one being measured are carefully positioned prior to the measurement, and do not change position during the measurement. *If the measurement includes movement from another joint, the results and conclusion will be flawed.*
- When measuring arms and legs, your back and pelvis should be as close to the neutral position as possible during the entire measurement to determine the ROM you have while the back is maintained in the neutral position.
- While evaluating your back ROM the PT notes the specific back positions that increase your pain, decrease your pain, and do not change your pain.

Certain motions are the most critical to your back during daily life, therefore the following range of motion measurements are recommended for the initial evaluation. This list is not intended for you to memorize, rather, it is provided so you have a better understanding of this approach and so you can judge if you've received the evaluation recommended in the System Limitations Approach to Pain.

Dorsiflexion with knee extension and the arch maintained in the foot.	(movement in the ankle joint pointing the foot up toward the knee,)
Calcaneal eversion	(heel moving out to the side)

Back in neutral prior to measurement:

Hip external rotation	(leg rolling out)
Hip internal rotation	(leg rolling in)
Hip abduction with knee extended	(leg moving out to the side, with knee straight)
Hip adduction with knee extended	(leg moving under the body, with knee straight)
Hip flexion	(hip bending while knee is bent)
Hip straight leg raise	(hip bending while knee is straight)
Hip extension (Thomas Test)	(hip straightening)
Shoulder flexion	(arm moving to overhead position from the front)
Shoulder abduction	(arm moving to overhead position from the side)
Shoulder internal rotation	(rolling shoulder in)

Standing, with no movement in the hips:

Trunk lateral flexion right	(standing, side bending right)
Trunk lateral flexion left	(standing, side bending left)
Trunk rotation right	(standing, upper trunk turning to right)
Trunk rotation left	(standing, upper trunk turning to left)
Trunk flexion	(standing, bending forward from the back)
Trunk extension	(standing, arching backward from the back)

Sitting, with no movement of the upper body:

Neck lateral flexion right

(bending head to the right side)

Neck lateral flexion left

(bending head to the left side)

Neck rotation right

(turning head to the right)

Neck rotation left

(turning head to the left)

Neck flexion

(bending head and neck forward)

Neck extension

(moving head and neck backwards, looking up)

Movements difficult to measure but important to note:

When lying on your back, note shoulder lift off the table (shortened pect minor)

Mid foot and forefoot motion (movement in the middle part of the foot)

Dropped 1st ray (the ball of the first toe is dropped down)

During the ROM measurements, it is extremely helpful for you to see and feel several examples of how limitations in your ROM cause your back to compensate during activities that increase your pain. As your back compensates for the limited ROM, some of you will actually experience your back pain increase during the ROM test. Understanding the effect of your limitations in this manner can serve as a great motivator to work on your program to improve your specific limited mechanics.

Motor Control: In the System Limitations Approach to Pain, the focus in the motor control part of the evaluation is your ability to control your back position while using your arms and legs for movement. The position I use to initially evaluate motor control is the same position I recommend for improving motor control in the Corrective Program. Lying on a firm surface such as the floor, use your trunk muscles to control your back in the neutral position while your legs perform an activity.

I believe that in this position your back has the best opportunity to demonstrate your motor control ability, for three reasons: 1) This is the easiest position for most people to put their back in the neutral position; 2) Gravity has the least effect on your trunk; and 3) The floor contact gives you feedback about your back position.

Your PT needs to consider all the Big Four Mechanics when deciding how to assess your motor control. Motor control is *not* a test of strength, although when your PT assesses your trunk control an inability to control your trunk might *reflect* a loss of strength. The inability to control your trunk might also *reflect* decreased range of motion if the test chosen requires range of motion that you do not have.

Strength: In this evaluation a manual muscle test (MMT) is used to determine the limitations in your strength. Some measurements test a specific muscle while other measurements test an action which includes a number of muscles. During a MMT the physical therapist positions your body and then asks you to perform the movement the muscle or muscles are responsible for. If you accomplish that movement, you hold a position at the end of the movement and the PT applies pressure. Your strength is determined by how far you can move and by how much pressure you can resist.

The test usually aggravates your pain this is why the MMT is usually delayed until a later time when it is likely to be less of a problem. I also try to schedule people for their MMT evaluations when they will have their best opportunity to recover; for example, on Friday just before the weekend.

Presently the MMT is graded on a scale of 0-5. In a 0/5 grade there is no activity of the muscle, such as when a muscle is paralyzed. In a 1/5 grade there is a flicker of muscle activity but it does not produce any movement. In a 2/5 grade the muscle contracts and moves the body part halfway through the motion which it is designed for. In a 3/5 grade the muscle contracts and moves the body part through the full motion but is unable to hold the position against any resistance. In a 4/5 grade the muscle contracts, moves the body part through the full motion, and then maintains that position against moderate resistance given by the PT. In a 5/5 grade the muscle contracts, moves the body part through the full motion, and then maintains that position against full resistance given by the PT.

If you demonstrate limited strength in the muscle or action you are testing, other muscles try to help and compensate for the limitation in strength. Testing can be very difficult when you have weaknesses that cause other muscles to compensate. Be relieved, not alarmed, if your PT brings out a manual muscle test book for reference during your test, this can help your PT sort out what your body is presenting and help adjust the test to your circumstances.

I believe it is important to look at the strength required for the activities that increase your back pain. For example, if it hurts to lift objects, you need to test the upper body strength that is required to perform the lifting, however, I do not often test the muscles of the lower back directly, due to the potential for aggravating the condition.

Additional Measurements: During your evaluation your PT might perform additional detailed measurements, including further ROM measurements, a sensation test, a joint play movement test, palpation of the soft tissue, special tests designed for the back, or other tests as your condition indicates.

ASSESSMENT

The assessment is the physical therapist's professional opinion of what is happening in your body, based on all the findings. The major determination in this assessment is whether the limitations identified in your body are related to the description of your pain.

To arrive at this assessment, your PT takes the following steps:

- Lists your mechanical limitations.
- Lists the activities that increase and decrease your pain.
- Lists the specific back positions that increase and decrease your pain.

When your limitations are related to your pain, your PT will explain as much of that relationship as possible.

Example (1):

You have a limitation in hip flexion range of motion (your hip bending to move the knee toward your chest).
Your pain increases when you sit.
Your pain increases when you move your back into the flattened position.
Assessment: Your back moves into the flattened position to compensate for decreased hip flexion when you sit. Therefore your hip limitation is related to your pain while sitting.

Example (2):

You have a limitation in hip extension range of motion (your hip straightening).
Your pain increases when you stand or walk.
Your pain increases when you move your back into the arched position.
Assessment: Your back moves into the arched position to compensate for decreased hip extension when you stand or walk. Therefore your hip limitation is related to your pain while standing.

Example (3):

You have a limitation in right hip adduction range of motion (right leg moving in under your body closer to left leg).

Your pain increases when you lie on your left side (right leg drops down toward left leg).
Your pain increases when you lean your trunk to the left (compensation for right hip adduction).
Assessment: Your back bends to the left to compensate for decreased right hip adduction when you lie on your side. Therefore your hip limitation is related to your pain when lying on your left side.

Some connections between your limitations and the activities that increase your pain are much more complex than these examples. You do not need to understand everything about mechanics and physical therapy; you only need to understand your body as much as you can, including the limitations you have and how they impact your back during activity. You will not understand everything at the time of the evaluation. The goal for you is to learn about and ultimately understand your body by the time you are finished with your PT.

Some of you are at a disadvantage in this process because you do not obtain immediate feedback from your back. When you change the position of your back, you do not get an immediate increase or decrease in pain. Although it is not as easy for you as for those who do have immediate feedback from pain, your PT can still determine if a relationship exists between your limitations and the activities that increase your pain.

If your PT doesn't find any mechanical limitations related to your back pain, your pain might not have a mechanical source. However, if you and your PT feel there is a mechanical aspect causing your back pain, you might need to keep asking questions and evaluating for possible missing information. Do not try to force a connection. If further evaluation does not reveal a connection, your PT should refer you to your physician for evaluation of other possible causes of your back pain.

PLAN

If the outcome of your evaluation is that you have mechanical limitations related to your pain, your PT will develop two programs, your Protective Program to protect your back and your Corrective Program to address your body's limitations. If indicated your PT will also plan additional treatment required to facilitate your progress.

Chapter 5 presents the details about the development of your Protective Program.
Chapter 6 presents the details about the development of your Corrective Program.

Your Additional Treatment: Your evaluation might reveal the need for additional treatment. Most of you will benefit from hands-on physical therapy to facilitate your progress. The hands-on physical therapy I use most often is joint mobilization and soft tissue work to help improve the mechanics. The joint mobilization I provide works in a gentle manner to increase the movement required inside each joint. The work on the soft tissue is directed at increasing the flexibility to improve the limited range of motion.

I recommend that physical therapists and other medical providers wait before providing any treatment that will decrease your pain until *after* you are able to decrease your pain on your own. Treatment that decreases your pain reduces your ability to learn from your pain, for example how to change an activity so you can do the activity without increasing your pain. I believe it is much safer to learn correct positioning and correct exercise technique when you have feedback from the pain. I also believe that it is much easier to ultimately achieve an exercise program that is not aggravating when you use the pain as feedback during the development of the exercise program.

Of course there are exceptions to this recommendation. There are cases where pain relief needs to be the primary focus. There are times when something during the session aggravates your pain, such as repeatedly trying exercise positions before finding one that is not aggravating. Your PT can then use manual therapy to minimize the chance of this activity increasing your pain.

RE-EVALUATION

In most cases your PT re-evaluates you informally at each session. A formal re-evaluation compares your present status with your initial status, focusing on the progress you make with your activity level, your mechanics, and your pain. You might not have re-measurements at every re-evaluation; this depends on your pain, how easily your pain is aggravated, and how long it has been since your last re-measurement. When you do not have re-measurements, a detailed, objective, and measurable description of your pain provides the important information about your progress.

Re-Measurements

Re-measurements are a part of the re-evaluation but are not a part of all re-evaluations. The re-measurements help evaluate how effective your exercises are at improving your mechanics. If your re-measurements demonstrate progress, you will continue your exercises until you reach your goals. If your re-measurements do not demonstrate progress, your PT will look at your exercise technique and how often you do the exercises to see if there are any problems with your present program and then make adjustments within an exercise or change some exercises altogether.

How Often?

Meet with your physical therapist at regular intervals for re-evaluation to discuss how your independent management is going, to demonstrate your exercise technique, and to assess how well you are progressing with your pain relief. Most PT regulations require a formal re-evaluation every month; however, for patients with long-term mechanical limitations that is too often. I believe that mechanical limitations do not change that quickly, and so monthly evaluations are costly and interfere with sessions to progress the program. Ultimately when you work on your own, the re-evaluation with re-measurements will occur every 12 weeks.

For most of you, the first re-measurements of your limitations will be 9-12 weeks after you complete the development of your initial exercise program. Further re-measurements will ideally be scheduled at 12-week intervals. You need time for the exercises to be effective, yet longer than 12 weeks is too long to do an exercise that is not working. During your re-measurements you might receive some or all of the testing you could not tolerate in the initial evaluation. Depending on how painful your back is and what your body tolerates, it might take several cycles of re-measurements before you complete the entire evaluation. For some in the RED group, repeated range of motion measurements might be too aggravating and therefore counterproductive. You might wait much longer than 12 weeks to have re-measurements.

Some of you in the RED or YELLOW group might be seen for physical therapy sessions in-between the re-measurements, for any additional physical therapy treatments you need to facilitate progress.

Continue with intervals of re-measurements until you and your physical therapist think you have maximized the development of your program and have progressed as far as you can with your mechanics. Many of you have had mechanical limitations for years, even decades, and, if you stick with your Corrective Program, you might continue making progress for years. If you have residual limitations, you might need to continue with your program to maintain your status while you await new ideas or new research to address your residual limitations.

Improvements

Based on the findings from your re-evaluation, you and your PT make appropriate changes in your plan. If your program is not complete your PT will likely add new stretches, new strengthening exercises, new postural activities, and new motor control activities. Your PT helps you take the next steps with your activity level, and provides manual therapy as indicated.

Improvements in your mechanics allow you to start or increase some activities. It is a challenge to sort out what you can and cannot start to do based on your progress; your PT will help you. Eventually you should learn how to increase your activity and simultaneously decrease your pain, on your own.

INFORMATION AND SUPPORT FROM YOUR PT

Think about any additional information you need from your PT. Do you understand his or her explanations? Are you getting enough information, in an organized way that you can absorb and use? Are you overwhelmed with too much information or explanations you cannot follow? Is anything getting in the way of your believing in your program and giving it all you've got? Do you feel the full support of your PT? Consider other kinds of support that could help you as well—for example, brainstorm with your PT what family and friends can do. How can you keep your motivation high? Do you do well with a list that you check off each day? Do you do well with a rewards system for sticking with your program? Give your PT feedback on what works well for you, and ask for changes that would be helpful to you. You are partners in this endeavor and the goal for both of you is your success.

Remember that what *you* do seven days a week has the biggest impact on your body. What your PT does in the office is a small part of your improvement program. You will be most successful when you understand your limitations and pain and fit your program into your life.

CHAPTER 5

Your Protective Program And Manual

OVERVIEW OF YOUR PROTECTIVE PROGRAM

Protect your back and decrease your pain

WHILE the ultimate goal is to improve your Big Four Mechanics as fully as possible, that can take months to years. Chapter 6, Your Corrective Program, explains that process. Meanwhile, you need to learn how to manage your back pain. The main goal of your Protective Program is to develop a plan to protect your back, by pursing the activities that decrease your pain and avoiding or modifying the activities that increase your pain.

The other goal is to develop a Quick-Relief Strategy to be able to decrease your pain on your own. The information you learn about your back positions while developing your Protective Program will also help you in the development of your Corrective Program.

Your program is built from information you gather during the steps in this chapter. The information you ultimately use to help you through your day will be found on Chart 2b and Chart 2c. Chart 2b is developed during Step 2b when you discover how you are positioning your back during activities that increase your pain. Chart 2c is developed during Step 2c when you learn how to modify everyday activities that increase your pain. To protect your back use the information from both charts to help you make choices about how to move through your day.

The Protective Program you build in this chapter is based on information about the back positions that increase your pain. Your PT will help you further build your program based on information about the back positions that decrease your pain. It would be too confusing to present both in one book.

You will use your pain as your guide to develop your Protective Program. Start by paying attention to what your back pain tells you. You already know a great deal about your back pain, and you may be consciously or unconsciously already taking steps to protect your back and decrease your pain. The more objective and detailed your awareness, the better decisions you and your PT can make for both your Protective and Corrective Programs. Writing down detailed, objective, measurable information about your pain will enable you to achieve the following goals:

- To identify if you have mechanical limitations that are contributing to your pain.
- To identify the specific back positions that cause your pain to increase and decrease.
- To identify the daily activities that cause your pain to increase and decrease.
- To create a customized Protective Program--a list of activities to pursue and avoid or modify and a quick-relief strategy to relieve pain in emergencies.
- To track your progress and to identify which parts of your program are effectively, efficiently helping you make progress.
- To create a Corrective Program with exercise positions that are least likely to increase your pain.
- To see measurable progress and stay motivated to continue your Protective and Corrective Programs.
- To communicate effectively with your PT by having objective and measurable information to discuss.

Summary

Following is the summary of steps you will take to develop your Protective Program:

STEP 1. DESCRIBE AND RECORD YOUR PAIN in as objective and measurable terms as possible. The more objective and measurable you can be, the better you will do.

STEP 2. PROTECT YOUR BACK

a) Identify and Record Your Best-Worst Back Positions. These are the specific positions of your back that increase, decrease, or do not change your pain.
b) Discover and Record the Relationships Between Your Activities and Back Positions. This step integrates Steps 1 and 2a to help you see how daily activities from Step 1 that increase and decrease your pain are related to the specific best and worst back positions from step 2a.
c) Plan and Record Your Helpful Positions. This step provides detailed information about how to approach typical daily activities. This step helps you learn positions to pursue, avoid or modify based on knowing the specific back positions that increase your pain.

STEP 3. RELIEVE YOUR PAIN: A QUICK-RELIEF STRATEGY.
You will identify a few positions and stretches that consistently decrease your pain, so that you know how to decrease your pain on your own.

Take your time

It will take time for you to truly understand how the activities that increase your pain are related to the specific back positions that increase your pain. If you rush through it, you risk learning only enough to decrease your pain while not learning enough to work on your long-term underlying problems.

Do not get frustrated if you cannot pursue the positions and activities that decrease your pain and avoid those activities that increase your pain every moment. If you try your best and shoot for performing your Protective Program 100 percent of the time, you will be successful 60-70 percent of the time and your back will be much happier.

General Activity Recommendations

CONTINUING ACTIVITIES YOU'VE BEEN DOING: Try not to eliminate activities. First try to modify an activity to perform it in a safe manner that allows you to protect your back and possibly help your back tolerate the activity without increasing the pain. Of course we are talking about reasonable and safe activities.

RESUMING ACTIVITIES YOU'VE STOPPED BECAUSE OF PAIN: Depending on your support system at work and at home, you might need to restart only activities that you know you can safely do every time. Until we change the culture around back pain, once you do something people usually think you can continue to do that activity every time. Patients often feel pressured, especially at work, to repeatedly perform an activity because some one saw them do the activity one time. If you can run up a hill once, that does not mean that you can safely run up the hill 20 times.

Also, wait to reintroduce an activity until you have a successful Quick-Relief Strategy and a full Corrective Program. If you reintroduce the activity too soon and your pain increases, it is difficult to know if the pain is increasing because of the new exercises or because of reintroducing the activity more rapidly.

STARTING NEW ACTIVITIES: If your pain increases, it can be difficult to know if it was the new activity or the new exercises in your Corrective Program. I recommend that you wait until you have both your Protective and Corrective Programs in place, with the ability to consistently decrease your own pain, before starting any new activities. Choose new activities wisely. Initially choose activities that you can perform in the best positions for your back.

RECORDING YOUR PERSONAL INFORMATION TO CREATE YOUR PROTECTIVE PROGRAM MANUAL

You should work on your answers to Step 1 prior to your PT evaluation. As you work through the rest of the steps with your PT, you can write down the information for each step, creating your own personal Protective Program Manual. Throughout this chapter are pages with charts and boxes designed for your information. You can copy these pages and create a separate manual; add as many blank pages as you need to fill in all the detail you can for each step. Or you can write your information down in the book. The following steps include instructions on how to fill out the charts and spaces provided for your information. Please read through the information and the detailed instructions before you start to write.

Writing the information down helps you further understand what you and your PT discuss and also creates a written record. The record helps you to: understand what is happening to your body, track your progress, identify problems in your program, make adjustments to your program, remember what to do when you have an episode of increased pain and stay motivated when you see how much progress you have made. So please spend the time *now* to gather and record as much information about your pain as possible.

WHY THE WRITTEN RECORD IS IMPORTANT

People in pain usually think they will remember the details of their pain without writing them down. Yet my experience is that most people forget many significant details about their pain.

One patient came to me with pain every time she drove. Her goal was to drive around town pain-free for five minutes. Three weeks after she started physical therapy she called reporting terrible pain after driving two hours. She sounded desperate. I asked how she felt for the first two hours and she responded that she was pain-free for the first two hours of the drive. When we discussed her five minute goal, she laughed and said, "Oh, I forgot!" When she realized how far she had come in three weeks she was no longer concerned and was in fact extremely pleased with her progress. Clearly she had made significant progress and should continue with the same program.

If we had not written down the initial status of her pain, I might have thought that there was a serious problem and changed her program. However, because of the written record I knew for sure that she had actually made great progress and that she should keep doing the program that was working so well.

Step 1. Describe And Record Your Pain

Complete as much of this step as you can prior to your PT evaluation. After the evaluation add any new information you learned. Pain can be difficult to describe. The six descriptors listed below provide language for you to describe your pain in detail, objectively, and measurably.

You will use a body diagram to provide the detail of the first three descriptors-location, size, and type of pain. You will then answer a list of questions that will help you describe in detail the last three descriptors-frequency, intensity, and duration of your pain. Your information will be written down in a series of charts. Associate the three descriptors with the activities you do prior to or during the time of the pain you describe. The frequency, intensity, and duration will be your primary way of communicating how you are doing to your PT.

WHY THE MEASURABLE DETAILS ARE IMPORTANT

Many people think they are describing their pain in a measurable and detailed way, yet are not being measurable or detailed enough. Following are two descriptions of an experience of pain, one in language that is general and other using measurable details. Following the initial descriptions is a progress statement. To see if there is a difference in the effect of information given, compare each initial statement to the progress statement and see if you can tell whether progress is made.

Initial Statement That's Too General: *Pain comes on after sitting awhile. The pain is a 0/10 when I wake up in the morning. The pain increases during the day to a 4/10.*

Initial Statement with More Measurable Details: *Pain comes on after sitting for approximately 15 minutes. Pain is 0/10 first thing in the morning. Around 10 a.m. the pain starts and is a 1/10. By 1 p.m. the pain is a 4/10.*

Progress Statement Three Weeks Later: *Pain comes on after sitting 45 minutes. Pain is 0/10 all morning, the pain starts around noon and by 4 p.m. the pain is a 4/10.*

Comparing the initial generalized statement to the progress statement does not suggest any progress. Comparing the initial statement with measurable details to the progress statement clearly demonstrates progress. If your descriptions are too general, you might not realize that you have made progress and you might change a program that is effective.

Often people use terms such as "awhile," "less pain," and "more pain" to describe their experience.

"Awhile" for one person could be fifteen minutes and "awhile" for someone else could mean two hours. *"I have less pain"* for one person could mean going from a 7/10 to a 6/10, and for another person it could mean a change from 7/10 to 2/10. Those experiences are very different. You need measurable language to record your initial situation and to communicate your experiences to your PT so that your PT can measure whether your program is working.

1A) BODY DIAGRAM TO DETAIL LOCATION, SIZE, AND TYPE OF YOUR PAIN

Instructions: Use the body diagram to describe, in detailed and measurable terms, the location, size and type of your pain. See Figure 5-1.

LOCATION: On the body diagram, outline the areas of pain and symptoms. If you have pain in more than one location, number them #1, #2, #3, and then refer to the number when describing the pain in that location.

SIZE: Use a measurable description of the size. *Five inches wide across the entire low back from right to left. A strip one inch wide down the outside of the thigh to the knee. A three inch wide strip down the outside of the thigh to the knee. The size of a quarter. The size of my fist. The entire foot, the bottom, top, inside and outside.*

TYPE: For each location describe the type of pain: *Aching, dull, stabbing, burning, shooting, throbbing, constant, intermittent, etc.* Identify areas of changes in sensation: *numbness, tingling, hypersensitivity.* Use any words you can think of to describe the type of your pain.

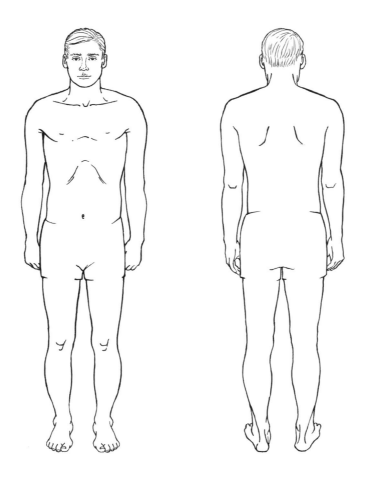

Fig. 5-1

1B) QUESTIONS TO DETAIL FREQUENCY, INTENSITY, AND DURATION OF YOUR PAIN

These three descriptors will serve as the monitors of your progress. To be helpful the frequency, intensity, and duration need to be associated with the activity you are doing around the time of the pain you are describing:

FREQUENCY of pain: How many days a week? How many times a day? How many times an hour?

INTENSITY of pain: Use a pain scale of 0-10, with 0 = no pain and 10 = worst pain.

DURATION of pain: How long does the pain last and how long are you pain-free? Try to use this language whenever describing increased or decreased pain with activity. For example: *Sitting is pain-free for 10 minutes, pain comes on after 10 minutes and if I continue to sit the pain increases. By 30 minutes of sitting the pain is a 7/10 and I need to get up. It takes 60 minutes to subside to a 2/10.* The duration can also be described as the percentage of the day you have pain: *100% of the day, 75%, 50%, etc.*

Here are two examples of detailed descriptions of pain:

> When I wake up at 7a.m. the pain in my left low back is a 1/10 and the size of a fist. The first 45 minutes of the day when I shower and get dressed my pain is a 1/10. When I drive to work the pain increased after 10 minutes to a 3/10. After 30 minutes of driving the pain increases to a 5/10. I have to move slowly to get out of the car. I have pain all day. I am never a 0/10. Most of the day the pain is a 5/10. However it increases to a 7/10 when I sit for more than 2 hours. The pain decreases about 3 times a day to 3/10. This happens when I am up and walking around for more than 20 minutes. When I get home at 6 p.m. the pain is a 7/10 and stays that way all evening until I go to bed.

> When I wake up at 7 a.m. my pain is a 2/10. It is painful all day. I am never a 0/10. The pain is an aching pain across my low back in a band about 5 inches wide. The pain goes up and down all day between a 2/10 and 9/10. It is difficult to know just how many times the pain changes—close to 20 times. The pain increases to a 6/10 when I stand for more than 10 minutes or walk for more than 15 minutes. The pain decreases to a 2/10 when I sit more than 10 minutes. When I get home from work the pain is a 5/10. It will stay that way all evening as long as I can limit walking and standing. If I go to an evening activity where I have to stand longer than 10 minutes the pain increases. If I stand more than an hour it increases to a 9/10. I do not know any way to decrease my pain other than to sit down.

WORST PAIN AND CIRCUMSTANCES:

Describe the worst pain you have had over the past two weeks—including frequency, intensity (on a scale of 0-10), and duration. What activity occurred just prior to that? If you do not know what increased your pain, note what activities you did an hour prior to that pain, during the earlier part of the day, and the night before. How often does this worst pain occur and how long does it last? What is the worst pain you have during a typical day (if different than the worst pain over the past two weeks)? What activity brings on the worst daily pain? How often does it happen during a day? How long does it last?

LEAST PAIN AND CIRCUMSTANCES:

Describe the least pain you've had over the past two weeks—including frequency, intensity (on a scale of 0-10), and duration. What activity occurred just prior to that? If you do not know what activity decreased your pain, note what activities you did an hour prior to that, during the earlier part of the day, and the night before. How often does this least pain occur and how long does it last? What is the least pain during the typical day (if different than the least pain in the last two weeks)? What activity occurs around the least daily pain? How often does it occur during the day? How long does it last?

Chart 1 Description of Your Pain (1 of 6)

Worst pain and circumstances:

Chart 1 Description of Your Pain (1 of 6)

Chart I Description of Your Pain (2 of 6)

Least pain and circumstances:

Chart I Description of Your Pain (2 of 6)

TYPICAL DAY:

Describe your typical day from the time you get up in the morning until the next morning. Use the following questions to help you be as detailed, objective, and measurable as possible. Describe in terms of frequency, intensity and duration. Make a note if the size changes.

- What is the intensity of your pain when you wake up in the morning?
- If you wake up pain-free, how long after you get up does the pain first start?
- If you wake up with pain, how long after you get up does the pain start to increase? or decrease?
- What are you usually doing at the time of day when the pain starts to increase?
- What do you do between getting out of bed and when the pain starts to increase?
- Once the pain increases how long does it last? Is there something you can do to make it subside? If there is something you can do, does it return to the level of pain just prior to the increase?
- If so, is that something you can do at work, school, or home?
- Describe the ups and downs of your pain each day.
- What levels of intensity of pain do you have during the day, on a scale of 1-10?
- How many times does the pain increase and decrease in a day? If you have so many ups and downs that it is difficult to know how many, guesstimate the number: 15, 25, 40 times?
- How long does each episode of increased pain last: Ten minutes? One hour? Until you stop the activity that increased the pain, for example sitting?
- If you have pain multiple times a day you may use a percentage to describe the amount of the day that you have a certain intensity of pain. How much of the day do you have pain? (25%? 50%? 100%?)
- What percentage of the day is your pain the worst?
- What percentage of the day is your pain the least?
- Does the most pain and the least pain come at a specific times each day?
- What is your usual pain intensity during the day on a scale of 0-10?
- Do you have a means to decrease your pain by yourself?
- Does the pain wake you at night? How many times? How long are you awake? Where is the pain? How intense is the pain on a scale of 0-10? Are you in the same position every time you wake up? Is there anything you can do to decrease the pain? (If so, note the position you take to decrease your pain: arch, flatten, bend to the right, bend to the left, or a certain leg position.)

If you have several typical days, describe each type of day noting the differences. You might note a difference between work days and the weekend, school days versus days off, or beginning of the week versus end of the week. You will further identify this in the description of your typical week.

Chart 1 Description of Your Pain (3 of 6)

Typical Day:

TYPICAL WEEK:

Most people do not have the same pain every day. In general, what is your week like?

- Consider your worst typical day of pain. How many days do you have like that in a week? What are you usually doing on those days?
- Consider your best typical day with the least pain. How many days do you have like that in a week? What do you do differently on these days?
- Is there a pattern to the days that you have your worst pain and least pain, e.g., beginning of the week? The day you have meetings all day?
- Do you have the same pattern every month? Do you notice seasonal pain (worse at the holidays or when gardening in the spring)?

OTHER SOURCES OF PAIN:

Add any other descriptions of pain you experience that are not described above. What pain do you have, for example, when you go camping, take care of the grandchildren, sleep in a hotel, etc.?

SPECIFIC DIFFICULT ACTIVITIES:

If you have specific activities that consistently increase your pain—for example, sitting, standing, walking, lying down, or driving a car—use this opportunity to describe them in detail. Provide as much measurable detail as possible, e.g., *if I sit for ten minutes and get up the pain goes away immediately; if I sit for more than thirty minutes the pain will last for 2 hours after I get up.*

Sitting: What kinds of chairs increase your pain more than others (soft or hard, high or low)? How long can you sit before the pain starts to increase? Do you move around a lot in the chair to try to prevent the pain from increasing? What sitting position do you assume to try to keep the pain as low as possible? Does it decrease right after you get up? If the pain lasts after you get up how long does it last?

Standing: How long before the pain starts to increase? Can you stand longer if you shift positions (e.g., lean up against a wall)? What can you do to make the pain subside? How long does the pain last after you stop standing position?

Walking: How long can you walk in distance or time before your pain comes on or starts to increase? How does terrain affect your pain, e.g. hills, uneven surface?

Driving in a car: How long do you drive before your pain starts? Or starts to increase? How long you can drive before you have to stop and get out? How long does your pain last after you stop driving? Do you make any changes to your seat?

Chart 1 Description of Your Pain (4 of 6)

Typical Week:

Chart 1 Description of Your Pain (5 of 6)

Other Sources of Pain:

Chart 1 Description of Your Pain (5 of 6)

Chart 1 Description of Your Pain (6 of 6)

Specific Difficult Activities:

STEP 2. PROTECT YOUR BACK

2a) IDENTIFY AND RECORD YOUR BEST-WORST BACK POSITIONS

While your whole body is in a position such as standing, sitting or lying down, your back has its own specific position. For example, when you are standing your back could be arched, neutral, flattened, bending to the right or left, or rotating to the right or left. I refer to these as your "specific back positions." While you perform activities during the day, you move your back through all these specific back positions. In this section you will move your back into all the specific back positions to see which are the best and worst for your back.

Your best positions are those in which you have your least back pain. They are also referred to as the most pain-free, or the positions that decrease your back pain. Your worst positions are those in which you have your most back pain. They are also referred to as the most painful, or the positions that increase your back pain.

The following information about best-worst back positions is also covered in the attached DVD.

When you have worked with your PT on your Best-Worst back positions and your PT has given you the okay to work on this more at home then follow the instructions and fill out the manual. Any instructions your PT gives supersedes these instructions.

FIRST READ THESE CAUTIONARY INSTRUCTIONS:

It is very important for you to read these Instructions *before* you try the back positions. Also watch the instructions on the DVD.

Only work on this after you have worked with your PT and they have told you can work on this on your own. You only work on this to re-enforce your understanding. Do not try this activity if you are in a lot of pain, if you have indications that your back is fragile, or if you will be upset if this activity aggravates your pain. In any of these cases wait until you are with your PT again. Being with your PT will not prevent this activity from aggravating your pain; it will provide you with professional advice to minimize the risk of increased pain.

Before starting, note if your back pain increases while sitting; if so, <u>flattening</u> your back probably increases your pain; see Figure 5-2a. If your back pain increases while standing and walking, <u>arching</u> your back probably increases your pain; see Figure 5-2b.

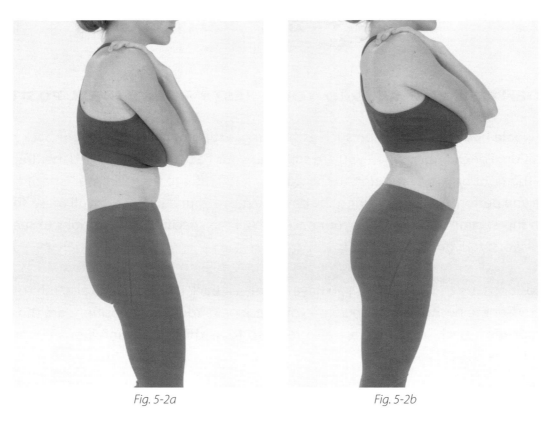

Fig. 5-2a   *Fig. 5-2b*

When you explore a position to see how it feels, do it only once or twice. The more repetitions you do the more likely you are going to aggravate your back. This is particularly important if you are in the RED group. If your back is presently in a painful flare up, and you cannot find any position of slightly decreased pain, wait and try again later in the day when your pain is not as angry, so that it can give you better feedback.

When you explore the specific positions, you will first move your back between arched and flattened. Somewhere in the movement between arched and flattened there will be a specific position where your pain is the most and another position where it is the least. See Figure 5-3. The specific positions of most or least pain could be (a) arched, (b) slightly arched, (c) neutral, (d) slightly flattened, or (e) flattened.

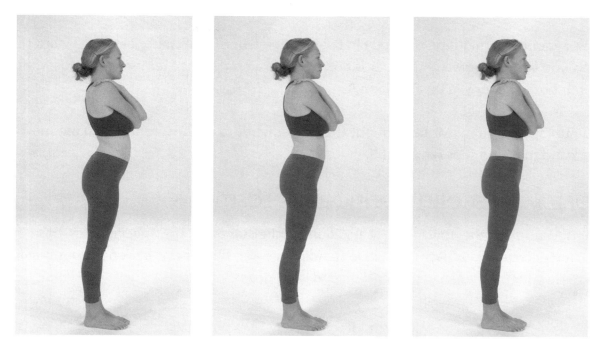

Fig. 5-3a   Fig. 5-3b   Fig. 5-3c

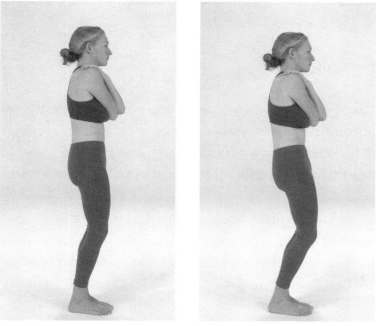

Fig. 5-3d   Fig. 5-3e

Look in the mirror. Your hips should be still. The movement should come from your back. To arch your back, gently stick your abdomen out in front. From the arched position slowly start to move your back toward the neutral position by decreasing the arch in your back, and then move to the flattened position by pulling your abdomen in and tucking your bottom under. First explore the back positions from arched to flattened once or twice to determine where your back pain is the most and least painful, or where there is no change in pain. Check the appropriate column in the chart, indicating your body's response to each of those specific back positions. Then explore the other specific back positions.

The rest of your body might be unhappy in the position where your back pain is the least. However, right now you are concerned with the position where your *back* is the least painful, not whether the rest of your body is happy in that position.

Continue to look in the mirror throughout the movements, to make sure that you are moving only your back and that your hips remain still.

EXPLORE AND RECORD SPECIFIC BACK POSITIONS

You will now explore the specific back positions while standing. The specific back positions that increase and decrease your back pain while standing are also the specific back positions that increase and decrease your pain when you are sitting and lying down.

Go ahead now and try this list of specific back positions in front of a mirror, and write down what you discover about your body in your manual chart that follows. For each specific back position, put an X on that line under the column "Worst Position," "Best Position," or "No Change." Add comments about the nature of your pain and the precise position such as slightly arched or slightly flattened. Use the form to describe what you experience.

Move through the following positions:

- Arch: Arch your back, with abdomen forward and bottom backward; see Figure 5-3a.
- Neutral: Given postural problems, you might not know your exact neutral in the beginning. Work with your PT to identify how neutral affects your pain.
- Flatten: Flatten your back, with abdomen sucked in and bottom tucked under; see Figure 5-3e.
- Side Bend right: Bend to the right, keeping your hips still; see Figure 5-4a.
- Side Bend left: Bend to the left, keeping your hips still; see Figure 5-4b.
- Rotate right: Rotate your upper body to the right, keeping your hips still and holding your arms across your chest; see Figure 5-4c.
- Rotate left: Rotate your upper body to the left, keeping your hips still and holding your arms across your chest; see Figure 5-4d.

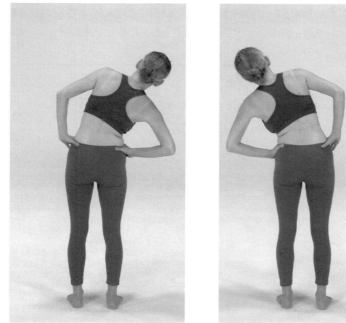
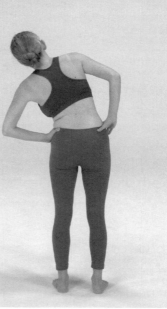

Fig. 5-4a   Fig. 5-4b

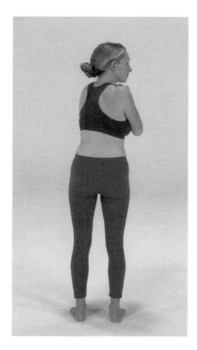
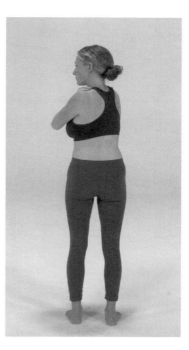

Fig. 5-4c   Fig. 5-4d

Chart 2a Best-Worst Specific Back Positions

Specific Back Position	Worst Position (most pain, or increases pain)	Best Position (most pain-free, least pain, or decreases pain)	No change	Comments
Arched				
Neutral				
Flattened				
Side Bend Right				
Side Bend Left				
Rotate Right				
Rotate Left				

2b) Discover and record relationships
between your activities and back positions

INTEGRATE STEPS 1 AND 2a

This is one of the most important steps in the whole program. It helps you identify relationships between the activities that increase and decrease your pain and the back positions that increase and decrease your pain.

It is the PT's role to review with you the specific back positions that *increase* your pain from Step 2a, and which painful activities from Step 1 use those painful back positions. You then repeat that process with the specific back positions and activities that *decrease* your pain.

You might find this process difficult if your answers in Step 1 are not very specific. If necessary, go back and fill in more detail in Step 1.

After you go through this step with your PT fill out the manual. The process of reading the instructions and writing your answers will help you further understand the relationship between the activities that increase and decrease your pain and the specific back positions that increase and decrease your pain.

The following are examples of relationships between *specific back positions* that increase pain and *activities* that *increase* pain:

- From Step 2a notes: Flattening is a specific back position that increases my pain.
- From Step 1 notes: Sitting at my desk and in the car increases my pain.
  Relationship: Sitting tends to flatten my back.
- From Step 2a notes: Arching my back is a specific back position that increases my pain.
- From Step 1 notes: My pain increases when I stand.
  Relationship: Standing tends to arch my back.
- From Step 2a notes: Bending to the right increases my pain.
- From Step 1 notes: My pain increases when I sit at my desk and reach into the desk drawers. All the drawers are on the right side of my desk.
  Relationship: Leaning to reach into the drawers causes my back to bend to the right.
- From Step 2a notes: Rotating to the left increases my pain.
- From Step 1 notes: My pain increases while I am at work. My office door is to the left of my desk and people come in all day.
- Relationship: Turning towards the door tends to rotate my back to the left.

The following are examples of relationships between *specific back positions* that decrease pain and *activities* that *decrease* pain:

- From Step 2a notes: Arching is a specific back position that decreases my pain.
- From Step 1 notes: My pain decreases when I walk.
  Relationship: Walking tends to arch my back.
- From Step 2a notes: Flattening is a specific back position that decreases my pain.
- From Step 1 notes: Sitting decreases my pain.
  Relationship: Sitting tends to flatten my back.
- From Step 2a notes: Bending to the right decreases my pain.
- From Step 1 notes: My pain decreases when I sit at my desk and lean on the right arm rest of my chair.
  Relationship: Leaning on the chair's arm rest bends me trunk to the right.

EXAMPLES OF POSITIONS AND ACTIVITIES

Chart 2b EXAMPLES consists of a list of specific back positions and next to it a box with activities that tend to use that particular specific back position. Everyone is different and activities will result in slightly different back positions for each of you. This is one of the reasons that you work with a physical therapist.

INSTRUCTIONS FOR FILLING IN *YOUR* CHART:

As you and your PT work on the specific back positions that *increase* and *decrease* your pain and the activities that use those positions, fill in your chart as much as you can. There is more room for the positions that increase your pain because as a rule there are more positions that increase pain than decrease pain.

To help you with this review your notes from Steps 1 and 2a.

- From your Step 2a chart, starting with the positions that increase your pain, write down one specific back position at a time in the left column.
- From your Step 1 notes and instruction from your PT identify the activities that use the specific back position you are focusing from Step 2a. Write those activities down in the right column on the chart in the box next to the corresponding box for the specific back position. Repeat this for every specific back position that increases your pain and every specific back position that decreases your pain.

Refer to Chart 2b EXAMPLES to help identify activities that might be related to your back pain. The information provided is just an example, there are additional activities you do each day to consider. You will not make a connection for *every* activity that increases and decreases your pain.

Chart 2b Example

From Step 2a manual notes: SPECIFIC BACK POSITIONS THAT CAN INCREASE or DECREASE YOUR PAIN	From Step 1 manual notes: EXAMPLES OF ACTIVITIES THAT OFTEN USE THAT SPECIFIC POSITION
Arched	• Standing • Walking on level surface • Walking up stairs and hills • Lying on your back with legs out straight • Reaching arms overhead
Flattened	• Sitting • Reaching forward or down • Bending forward • Bringing your knees to your chest (e.g., putting on shoes & socks) • Lying on your side with knees and hips bent or curled up
Bent to the left or right	• Leaning to the side to pick up purse or bag • Emptying dishwasher • Working in drawers at side of desk • Carrying something heavy on your side like backpack, child • Sometimes walking
Rotated to the left or right	• Turning to talk to someone when sitting or standing at meals or meetings • Throughout household and work activities, pay attention to the times you rotate your upper body in relation to your lower body

Chart 2b Your Chart

From Step 2a	From Step 1
Specific Back Positions that increase your pain	Activities that use that position that increase your pain
Specific Back Positions that decrease your pain	Activities that use that position that increase your pain

2c) Plan and record your helpful positions

INTRODUCTION:

In Step 1, Describe and Record Your Pain, you created a detailed, objective, and measurable description of your pain, including activities that increase and decrease your pain. In Step 2a, Identify and Record Your Best-Worst Back Positions, you identified specific back positions that increase and decrease your pain. In Step 2b, Discover and Record Relationships between Your Activities and Back Positions, you learned about the relationship between your daily activities and the specific back positions that increase and decrease your pain.

In Step 2c specific recommendations are given about how to approach everyday activities. You are given recommendations of what to pursue and what to avoid based on information about the specific back positions that *increase* your pain.

The activities that increase your pain can be modified and if they no longer increase your pain then they become activities to pursue. Hopefully you can avoid the reason for the increased pain during a specific activity and then not have to avoid the activity altogether.

The recommendations are specified for six pain patterns. From the pattern's description, determine if it applies to you. You need to follow only the recommendations for the patterns that apply to *your* pain.

Not all the recommendations will work for everyone. Try not to get frustrated as you and your PT test what works for your body. Keep in mind that a position that decreases your pain will not necessarily decrease it 10 out of 10 times; it might help 7-8 out of 10 times.

As your mechanics improve and you learn to control your back position, you will find that you can move activities up your chart from activities to avoid to becoming activities you can pursue.

The following information about helpful positions is covered in the attached DVD.

PATTERN 1: PAIN INCREASES WHEN YOU ARCH YOUR BACK

In this pattern your pain increased in Step 2a when you arched your back. In general, your pain increases when you stand, walk (especially when you walk up stairs or hills), or lie down on your back with legs out straight. Your pain usually decreases when you sit or lie down with hips and knees bent. *If this description fits you, try the following suggestions:*

Standing:

<u>Avoid</u> standing for prolonged periods of time, and avoid standing in shoes with high heels.

- High heels force your back into an increased arch; see Figure 5-5. If you are accustomed to wearing high heels your calf muscles might be tight and short, so you might need to compromise at first by wearing shoes with lower heels rather than flat heels. Wearing a lower heel will help care for your back, and keeping some heel will help compensate for the tight calf muscles until you are able to stretch your calf muscles enough to allow a better foot position with flat heels.

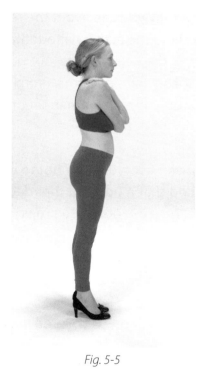

Fig. 5-5

<u>Pursue</u> standing with a decreased arch in your low back. Try the following strategies:

- Put a foot up on a low stool; see Figure 5-6.

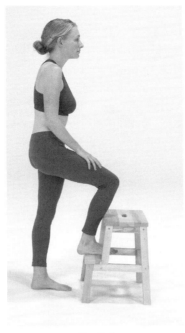

Fig. 5-6

- Prop your bottom on a counter top or barstool-height chair; see Figure 5-7.
- Lean your back up against a wall with a slight bend in your hip and knee.
- Bend one knee and set the knee down on the seat of a chair; see Figure 5-8. The taller you are, the higher the chair you need for this.
- Tuck your bottom under and slightly bend your knees if you need to; see Figure 5-9. This is difficult to maintain, but you can do it for a short time to get a little relief.

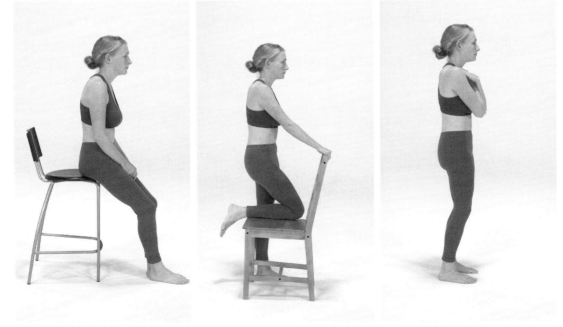

Fig. 5-7   *Fig. 5-8*   *Fig. 5-9*

Sitting:

<u>Avoid</u> a firm chair that is too high for your feet to touch the floor; see Figure 5-10. When your feet do not touch the floor, the arch in your back usually increases.

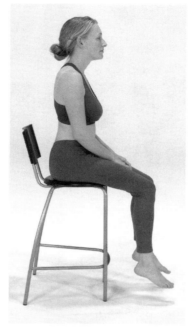

Fig. 5-10

<u>Pursue</u> sitting with your feet supported so that your knees are higher than your hips. Here are a few strategies to move your back out of the arch and move towards a flattened position:

- Sit in a low chair, with the seat at or below your knee level; see Figure 5-11.
- Use a bucket seat in a car.
- Choose a low or medium height chair with a lot of cushion.

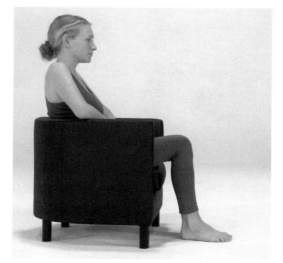

Fig. 5-11

- Choose a chair with a railing and put your foot on the rail; see Figure 5-12.

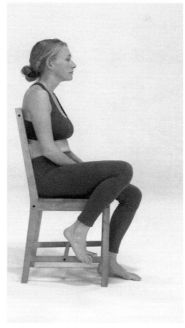

Fig. 5-12

- Sit with your feet up on a stool or ottoman, as in Figure 5-13.

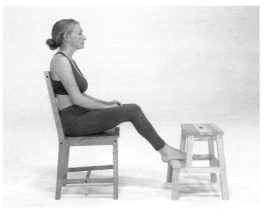

Fig. 5-13

Lying Down:

<u>Avoid </u>lying in a way that is likely to increase the arch in your back; for example:

- Lying on your stomach; see Figure 5-14.
- Lying on your side with an arch in your back.
- Lying on your back with your legs out straight, as in Figure 5-15.

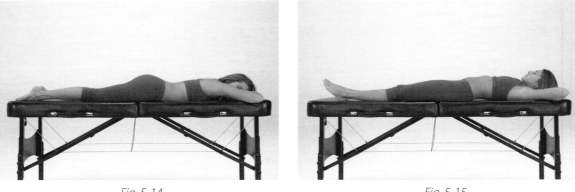

<table>
<tr><td>Fig. 5-14</td><td>Fig. 5-15</td></tr>
</table>

<u>Pursue</u> lying in a way that flattens your back.

- Lie on your back with pillows under your knees. If you have a large arch in your back, put several pillows under your knees; see Figure 5-16.
- Put your legs over two couch cushions when you are in a lot of pain or if you need that to decrease the arch in your back; see Figure 5-17.

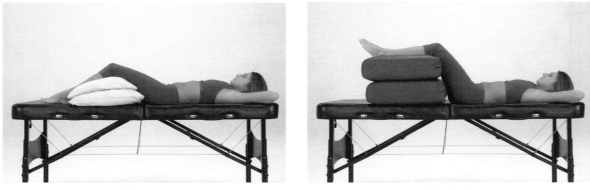

<table>
<tr><td>Fig. 5-16</td><td>Fig. 5-17</td></tr>
</table>

- (This position is demonstrated on the DVD) When lying on your side bend your hips and knees to a point where you feel your back is in its best position, not too arched or too flattened. Put two or more pillows between your legs between your knees and feet. Some of you might need to make sure your leg is above hip height in order to decrease your pain. The foot should be well supported on the pillow and not drop off the edge. Try pillows with and without the feet supported and see the difference in how well supported you feel. If you have a small waist and/or broad shoulders, you might feel better with a small pillow under your side. The pillow needs to be very small like an infant pillow, and soft; otherwise it could put uncomfortable pressure on your side. When lying on your side a pillow for your head needs to be thick enough to fill the space between your ear and shoulder.

Reaching Up:

<u>Avoid</u> reaching up and allowing your back to arch when you reach. For example:

- Reaching for objects off a high shelf, as in Figure 5-18.
- Reaching up into cabinets for dishes or food.
- Taking off a sweatshirt or washing hair.

<u>Pursue</u> reaching what you need in ways that keep your back flattened or neutral.

- Raise yourself up on a stepstool so that the object is not above shoulder height.
- Adjust your environment to minimize having to reach up; for example, move your coffee mug and any other frequently used dishes from the cabinet to the counter; move clothes to a lower shelf, as in Figure 5-19. Reaching to a level between your shoulder height and hip height is most likely to keep your back in its most neutral or pain-free position.
- Prior to all reaching-up activities, tuck your bottom under to decrease the arch in your back; see Figure 5-20.

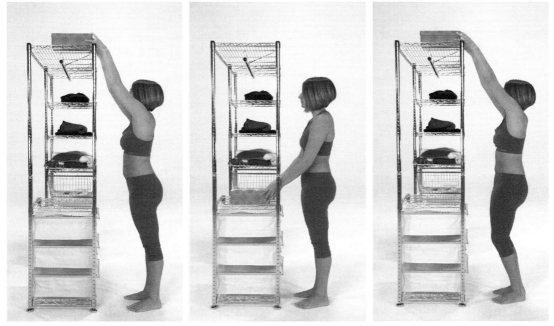

Fig. 5-18   *Fig. 5-19*   *Fig. 5-20*

Walking:

<u>Avoid</u> long step lengths, because the farther your leg moves behind your body the more your back arches, which can increase your pain; see Figure 5-21.

<u>Pursue</u> short step lengths, and if possible tuck your bottom under slightly to decrease the arch in your back; see Figure 5-22.

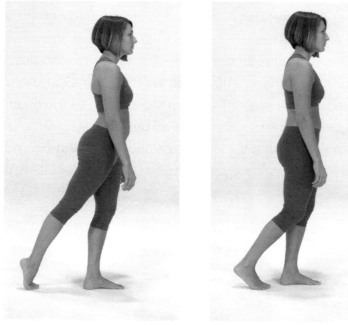

Fig. 5-21   Fig. 5-22

PATTERN II: PAIN INCREASES WHEN YOU FLATTEN YOUR BACK

In this pattern your pain increased in Step 2a when you flattened your back. In general, in this pattern your back pain increases with one and/or all of the following positions: sitting, bending, reaching forward, reaching down, and bringing your knees toward your chest. Your pain might decrease when you stand, walk, or lie down on your back. *If this description fits you, try the following suggestions.*

Standing:

This is not usually a problem for people whose pain increases when they flatten their backs. You needn't avoid standing, and you might want to pursue walking.

Reaching Down:

<u>Avoid</u> reaching down in a way that flattens your back.

- Reaching below waist level with both legs straight tends to flatten your back; see Figure 5-23.

<u>Pursue</u> bringing your activity up to waist height so you do not have to reach down; see Figure 5-24.

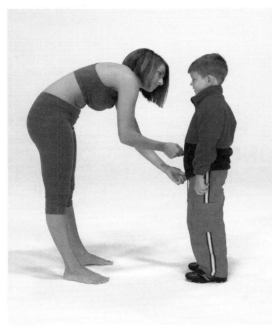

Fig. 5-23

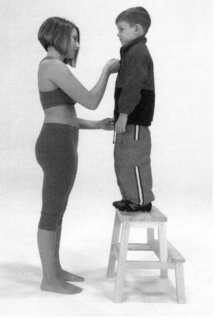

Fig. 5-24

<u>Pursue</u> reaching down below waist level in ways that minimize flattening your back:

- Use a golfer pick-up position, with one leg raised behind you; see Figure 5-25.
- Squat down, bending your hips and knees; see Figure 5-26.
- Use a reacher to extend the reach of your arm, as in Figure 5-27.

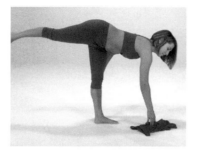
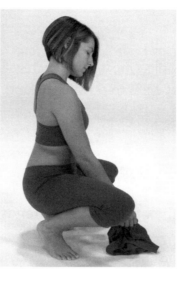
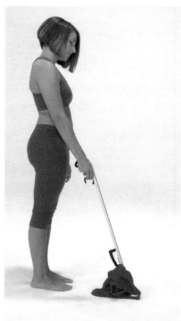

Fig. 5-25   *Fig. 5-26*   *Fig. 5-27*

SAFE ZONE

Note that reaching above shoulder height tends to arch your lower back, and reaching below waist level tends to flatten your lower back. Activities between shoulder and waist levels do not tend to move your back much unless you have significant loss of trunk strength and stability.

Sitting:

Avoid low seats, bucket seats and chairs with a lot of cushioning. These chairs tend to put you're your back in the painful flattened position; see Figure 5-28.
A low seat is one that is below your knee joint height when you stand next to it.

Avoid bringing your knee towards your chest while sitting.

Pursue firm, high chairs, with a seat above your knee height. They do not let your back flatten as much as low, soft chairs do. A chair in which your feet do not touch the ground can actually help move your back out of the flattened position; see Figure 5-29.

Pursue chairs with backs that recline, so that the hip does not have to bend to a full 90 degree angle. You can lean the seat back to decrease the amount of bend you need to sit. This will increase the chance that the bend will come from your hip rather than from your back, helping your back to stay in the neutral position. Examples are computer chairs, as in Figure 5-30, executive chairs and recliners.

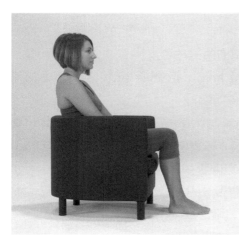

Fig. 5-28

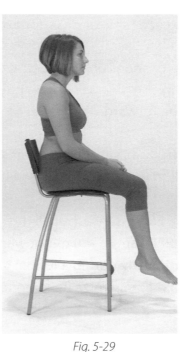

Fig. 5-29

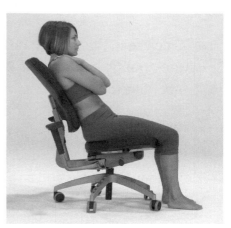

Fig. 5-30

DIFFERENT MECHANICS IN EACH HIP

You might find that your back pain only decreases when your hips are in two different positions. For example, you might have less pain when one hip is bent and the other hip is straight. In this case you might find that when you lie down you bend one leg and bring it close to your chest, while you keep the other leg straight. Or you might find that when you lean back in a reclining chair that one leg is ok when straight but the other leg needs to be bent.

Reaching Forward:

<u>Avoid</u> any forward trunk motion that moves your chest toward your knees because it might flatten your back. Here are some examples of what to avoid:

- Reaching forward when sitting at a table or desk, for example to reach for the phone, as in Figure 5-31.
- Reaching forward to put socks or shoes on your feet.

<u>Pursue</u> strategies to minimize reaching forward.

- Sit close to the table or desk in a firm, supportive chair, as in Figure 5-32.
- Pre-arrange items on the desk so that frequently-used items are in arm's length and you do not have to reach.
- Plan ahead at the dinner table. For instance, put all the items you want on your plate prior to sitting down. If you are in the RED range, you might want to ask your family members to help you reach what you need, particularly during a formal dinner setup.
- Use slip-on shoes and a sock aid to minimize needing to bring your knees toward your chest.

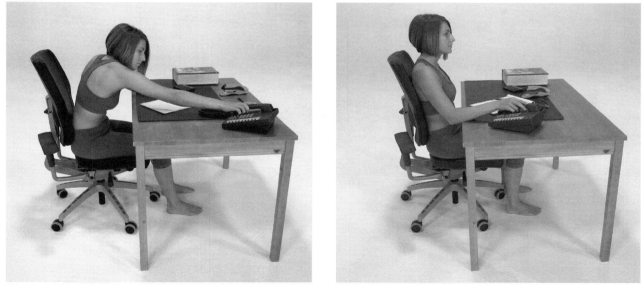

Fig. 5-31 Fig. 5-32

Lying Down:

<u>Avoid</u> bringing your knees towards your chest so that it flattens your back.

- Lying down on your back on a soft couch, in a hammock, or in a very soft bed generally causes the back to move into a painful flattened position. In Figure 5-33, the position in the hammock demonstrates what tends to happen in a soft bed or soft couch.
- Lying on your side curled up with your knees and hips bent tends to flatten your back.

<u>Pursue</u> positions that move your back toward neutral or slightly arched.

- Lying on your back on a firm bed or couch with your legs out straight. In the short run, you might be more comfortable with a small pillow under your knees, Figure 5-34.

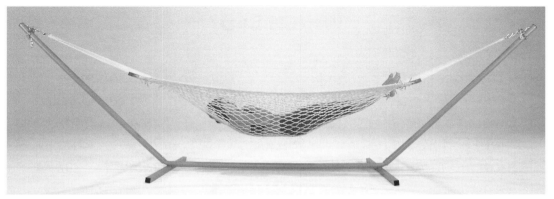

Fig. 5-33

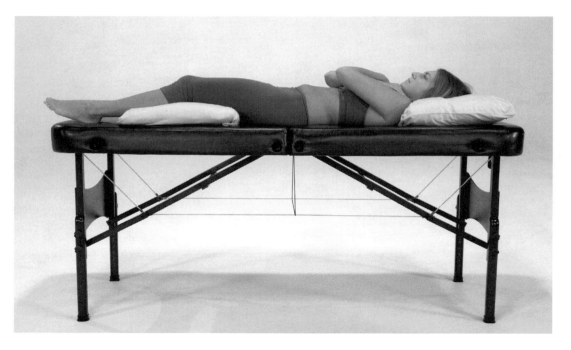

Fig. 5-34

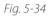

- (This position is demonstrated on the DVD) For your best position when lying on your side, put two pillows between your knees and feet. Move your back out of the flattened position and into your most pain free position. The top foot should be well supported on the pillow and not drop off the edge of the pillow. Some of those in the RED group might need 3 pillows between your legs to bring the top leg to or above hip height. Try pillows with and without the foot supported and see the difference in how well supported you feel. For some of you, especially if you have a small waist and/or broad shoulders, your back might feel better supported with a small pillow under your side. The pillow needs to be very small like an infant pillow, and soft; otherwise it can put uncomfortable pressure on your side or ribs.

WHICH BED?

The right kind of bed for you depends on what position makes your pain better or worse. If you prefer your back flattened, you would do best in a soft bed. If you prefer an arched position, a firm bed would be best for you. Of course your other mechanical limitations can alter the situation considerably. The only way to know if your back tolerates a bed is to try sleeping in it repeatedly for a period of time.

PATTERN III: PAIN INCREASES BOTH WHEN ARCHING AND WHEN FLATTENING

A number of people have pain that increases both with arching and with flattening. If you are one of those people, look at the two previous pattern descriptions for what to avoid. In Pattern I concentrate on the information about standing and lying down, and in Pattern II concentrate on the information about sitting, reaching down, and reaching forward.

Regarding what to pursue, ideally there is a spot between arched and flattened where you have no pain or at least minimal pain. Explore moving from arched to flattened to discover the position where the pain is the least. If you are in a lot of pain do not repeatedly explore the back positions during any one session, since that can really aggravate your back. If you do not get enough information when you explore the positions 1-2 times, try it again later in the day. Once you identify the position of least pain, work to achieve that specific back position of decreased pain while standing, sitting, and lying down. You might need to slightly vary the position of your legs to achieve this position.

PATTERN IV: PAIN INCREASES WHEN YOU BEND TO THE SIDE

In this pattern, the pain occurs on the side you bend *toward*. If you have a sensation on the side you bend away from, it is probably a stretch sensation that should subside with gentle stretching. If it continues, have that area evaluated.

<u>Avoid</u> bending toward the side that hurts. For example:

- Bending to the painful side when putting an item down on the floor, like a computer bag or a purse, as in Figure 5-35.
- Holding heavy objects like children, groceries or backpacks over one arm on the painful side.

<u>Pursue</u> bending away from the painful side.

- Put objects down on the other side so that you bend away from your painful side; see Figure 5-36.
- Hold children, back packs, or groceries on the side away from the pain.
- Keep a slight bend away from the pain when sitting or standing. You might find it helpful to rest on the non-painful side with your arm on an arm rest, counter or table.

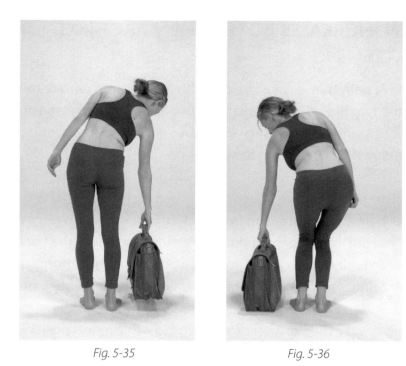

Fig. 5-35   *Fig. 5-36*

PATTERN V: PAIN INCREASES WHEN YOU ROTATE YOUR BACK

As with side-bending, if rotation to one side increases pain, rotation to the other side usually has no effect on the pain or decreases the pain. Full rotation to the end of the motion in both directions can increase pain for some in the RED and YELLOW groups.

Avoid rotating your upper body toward the side that increases the pain.

Avoid sitting or standing in a position that requires you to rotate in the painful direction. For example:

- Turning to talk to people, as in Figure 5-37.
- Listening to a presentation or helping a child; see Figure 5-38.

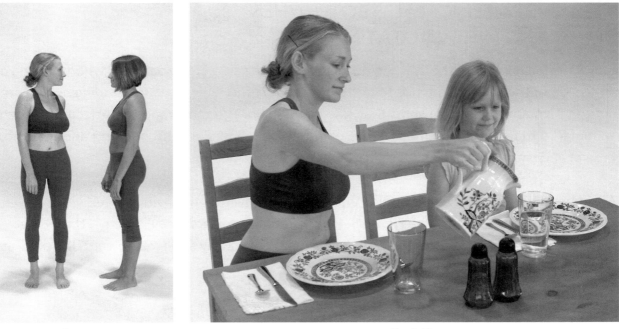

Fig. 5-37   Fig. 5-38

<u>Pursue</u> positions that do not require you to rotate your upper body toward the painful side.

- Turn your entire body towards the activity, as in Figure 5-39.
- Set up your office, kitchen, bedroom, bathroom, or any place you work regularly in a way that limits the times you must rotate your upper body to the painful side.
- If rotating to one side decreases the pain, then slightly rotate in that direction when possible.

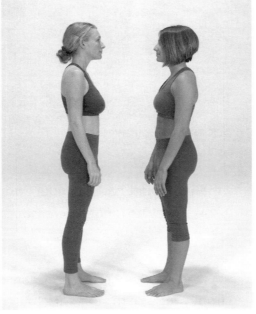

Fig. 5-39

PATTERN VI: PAIN INCREASES BOTH WHEN BENDING AND WHEN ROTATING

In many cases pain increases both when *bending toward* the side of the pain and when *rotating away* from the side of the pain. Pain tends to *decrease* with just the reverse, when *bending away* from the side of the pain and *rotating towards* that side of the pain. The movement that decreases the pain is a minimal to moderate movement in the pain-free direction. For both bending and rotating, the extreme of each movement in either direction will probably increase the pain.

> <u>Avoid</u> bending toward the painful side and rotating away from the painful side.
>
> <u>Pursue</u> bending away from (see Figure 5-40) and rotating toward (see Figure 5-41) the side with pain. A short line to remember what to pursue is "lean away and twist toward" the pain, as in Figure 5-42.

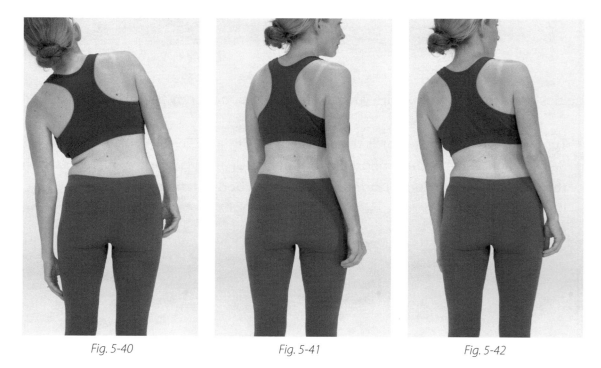

Fig. 5-40   Fig. 5-41   Fig. 5-42

INSTRUCTIONS FOR CHART 2c

After reading the descriptions and recommendations for each pattern, write the positions that increase your pain and details about them in your Chart 2c under Positions to Avoid. Try the positions that are recommended for you to pursue. If they no longer increase your pain write them down under Positions to Pursue.

Following Chart 2c are Additional Tips which include recommendations for moving from lying down to sitting and sitting to lying, rolling from your side to your back and from back to side, getting in and out of the car, when driving, and when sitting at a computer. Review all this with your PT and based on your needs, list in Chart 2c what fits you to avoid/modify and pursue from these tips as well.

Chart 2c Planning Your Helpful Positions

Positions to Avoid	Details

Positions to Pursue	Details

ADDITIONAL TIPS TO DECREASE PAIN WHILE MOVING

Moving from lying down to sitting: Protect your back by first moving your back into the neutral or most pain-free position. For most of you that will mean that you bring your knees and feet toward your trunk by bending your hips and knees, as in Figure 5-43. Once you are in the neutral or least painful position, log roll on to your side, keeping your neutral back position. From your side, slide your feet off the edge of the bed, and then use both hands to push up to sit as your legs lower down, (see Fig. 5-44), again keeping your back in its neutral and most pain-free position; see Fig. 5-45.

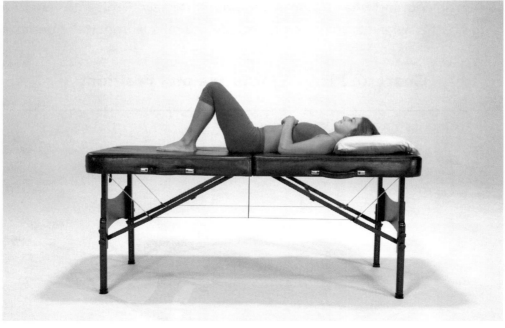

Fig. 5-43

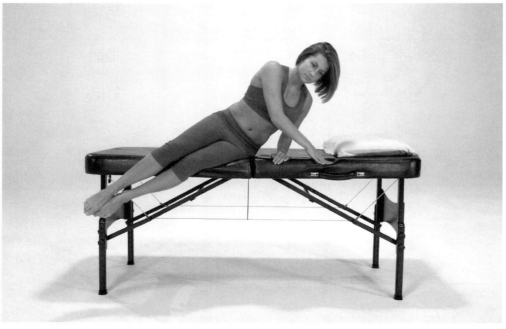

Fig. 5-44

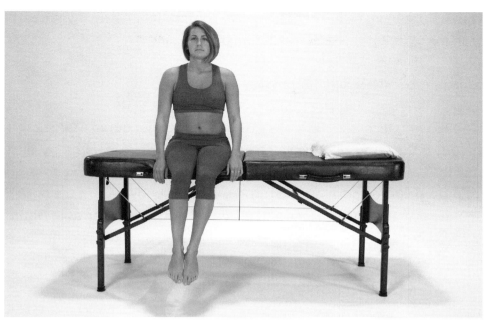

Fig. 5-45

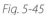

Moving from sitting to lying down: To lie down, do the above in reverse. Keep your back in its neutral or most pain-free position and use your hands to walk your trunk down on to your side on the bed, bringing your feet up at the same time; see Figure 5-44. You end up lying on your side on the bed. Keeping your knees bent, log roll onto your back, as in Figure 5-43. Keep your back in its neutral or least-painful position throughout the activity.

Adjusting bed pillows when moving from lying on your side to lying on your back: When using a number of pillows for positioning, it is good to plan ahead on how to change positions, in order to minimize your back movement and aggravation. Take any pillows out from under your side. Make sure your back is in your neutral or most pain-free position and that it stays there throughout the activity. The easiest move for your back is to use your feet to move the pillows from between your legs to under your knees. Log roll from your side onto your back. If needed, change the pillow under your head from a larger one that keeps the neck in neutral when on your side to a small pillow that better supports your head when you are on your back.

Adjusting bed pillows when moving from lying on your back to lying on your side: Reversing this movement takes a little more effort to position the pillows. If needed, position a pillow under your side before you roll (refer to the DVD). Reach down and take the pillows from under your knees. Roll onto your side and slide the pillows between your legs. If needed, change the head pillow to a thicker or second pillow to adequately support your neck on your side.

Riding in a car: Consider two main challenges when riding or driving in a car: getting in and out of the car and your position in the car. Strategize your approach to both challenges with your physical therapist. Together you can determine what adaptations to try. Take into account your best back positions, your specific mechanical limitations, and the design of your car.

Consider the following specifics with your physical therapist:

A) Getting In and Out: Of course it is easier on your back to get out of a large car than a small car. The technique is the same whether you have a small, medium, or large car. First, <u>avoid</u> stepping out of the car to stand up on one leg, as in Figure 5-46. Instead, keep your back in your neutral or most pain-free position and turn your whole body toward the door. You end up sitting on the car seat with both feet on the ground outside the car, as in Figure 5-47. From that position, scoot your bottom to the edge of the seat, put one hand on the back of the car seat and the other hand on a safe and non-moving part of the car and use both hands to support you while you stand up; see Figure 5-48.

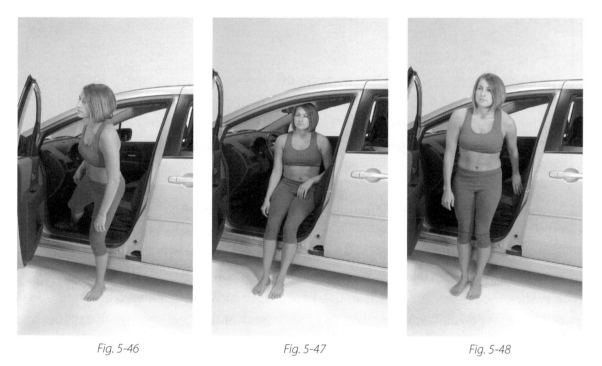

Fig. 5-46   Fig. 5-47   Fig. 5-48

To get in the car, follow the instructions above in reverse. Sit down on the edge of the car seat, slide your bottom back on the seat, and then bring one foot in at a time while you turn your body to the front of the car, keeping your back in its neutral or most pain-free position throughout the motion.

B) Your Position in the Car

1. Is it a bucket seat? From a standing position next to the driver's side with the door open, squat down and look at the side of the seat, or have someone do it for you. Most cars have a significant bucket seat, which means that the seat bottom slopes down in the back and

raises up high at the knees. Whether this is good or bad depends on what you need. For those of you who want to flatten your back, this is good. For those of you whose back pain increases with flattening, you will need to make some adjustments. Some cars have the mechanism to lift up the back of the seat and lower the front. Try that while you are sitting in the car. If you do not have that feature, you can add some towels in layers until the seat is more level. Do not do this if raising you up affects your visibility, for example, puts your eye level so that the rearview mirror obstructs your view. This also does not work for a tall person in a low car, because it raises you too close to the ceiling.

2. Are there wedges or rolls on either side on the seat running alongside your leg? The problem with the wedges or rolls is that it limits your ability to set your leg out to the side. This is a problem for those of you who have a limitation in hip adduction where the lack of hip adduction motion affects your back position and so you want to set your leg out to the side. This does not mean just rolling your knee out; it means picking up your entire thigh off the seat and setting it to the side. You will discover whether hip adduction is a problem for you during your System Limitations Evaluation. The physical therapist measures your hip adduction at that time and determines if a limitation there matches your pain.

3. If this is a problem for you, the fix is to fill in the seat to make it level between the wedges. As above, some of you cannot fill in the seat because it would raise you up too high affecting your visibility, your head might touch the ceiling or the rear view mirror might block your view.

4. What is the structure of the seat back? The back of the seat needs to support your back in your neutral or most pain-free position. Most cars have a lumbar roll to support the arch in your low back; however, for many people it is not the right size or in the right spot. And the upper part of the seat back often sinks too far back.

5. How high is the seat from the floor? Seats that are high up off the floor as in SUV's and mini-vans give you the option to position your back in its neutral or most pain-free position. Seats that are low to the floor tend to flatten your back.

Working at a computer: Work to achieve the position in Figure 5-49. Start positioning from the ground up. First make sure your feet are fully in contact with the floor. An inclined board is often recommended for the foot position; however, very few people actually use an inclined board. Adjust the seat of your chair to the height at which your knee bends at a 90 degree angle. This positions your thigh parallel to the floor. Position the back of your chair to support your back upright, with a 90 degree angle at your hips and with your pelvis level. (The back of the chair will not actually be *completely* upright since that would tilt most of you forward. The chair back should ideally be reclined slightly back from 90 degrees.) It should ideally support your neutral back position with a slight arch in your back. If you have a high back chair you want the curve in the upper part of the chair to support your upper back in neutral position. Your forearms should rest on the arm rest in a position that is parallel to the floor. The height of any arm rest should position the shoulders at shoulder height and not force the shoulders up towards your ears higher than shoulder height, or drop your shoulders lower than shoulder height. The keyboard should be at the level of your forearms. The top of the computer screen should be at eye level.

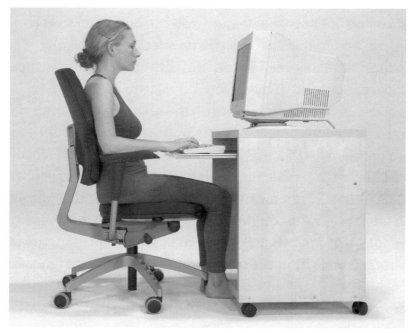

Fig. 5-49

STEP 3. RELIEVE YOUR PAIN: A QUICK-RELIEF STRATEGY

3a) INTRODUCTION

The Quick-Relief Strategy is a way for you to have some control over your pain and be able to decrease your pain on your own if you happen to have an episode of increased pain. This strategy is made up of two to four positions and/or stretches that decrease your pain most of the time, I want you to have your Quick-Relief Strategy *before* you start the exercises in your Corrective Program. That way if you start an exercise that turns out to aggravate your back or overdo an exercise or home activity, which almost everyone does at least once, you are not stuck at home with increased pain; you can do something on your own to decrease your pain.

Many of you might need to use the Quick-Relief Strategy after you feel your best, as many people feel their worst pain after they feel their best. What usually happens is that you feel really good, with no sign of back pain and no guarding from the pain. If you feel that way you might engage in an activity or multiple activities that turn out to be too much and your pain returns. You can then use your Quick-Relief Strategy to decrease your pain.

I hope you use your Quick-Relief Strategy for its intended purpose and not to enable you to continue to do activities that you know increase your pain. Continuing to engage in painful activities without first addressing your mechanical limitations can cause further aggravation to your back.

To find positions and stretches for your Quick-Relief Strategy, you and your physical therapist will note the level of your pain prior to and after trying different positions and stretches. Together you select the positions and stretches that most consistently decrease your pain. Then plan how you can do at least two of them in each of your environments, e.g., home, school, or work.

Write your Quick-Relief Strategy down in your Manual pages that follow the suggestions below. Barring any unforeseen accident or new problem, this will continue to be the strategy that decreases and/or manages your back pain while you address your mechanical limitations.

3b) USE ACCORDING TO YOUR GROUP

REDS: For those of you in the RED group, your Quick-Relief Strategy might include alternating from one best position to another. When you are in a lot of pain even your best position is only helpful for a limited time. So what do you do? You learn how long a position is helpful before your pain starts to increase, and you switch from position to position *before* your pain starts to increase. For example, you find that your pain increases after 20 minutes in your best position. You know what your three best positions are and the most pain-free way to move from position to position. You start in one position such as lying on your side; after 18 minutes you move to lying on your back; after 18 minutes you move to your best seated position; after 18 minutes you move back to the side position. If you continually change positions to your next least painful position, you might find that you can reduce your pain.

You will probably find the most helpful positions to be the floor clock, a side-lying position in bed, a reclining position in a chair, and a couple of stretching positions such as the half knee stretch or the seated low back stretch.

YELLOWS: If you are in the YELLOW group, you might occasionally need to alternate between positions to decrease the pain as described above for the RED group. This could happen on a day when you overdo activity or participate in some unexpected event. For the most part you will use several stretches and just one position to decrease your pain. Unless you are close to being a RED you will probably only need one reclining position such as the floor clock or a reclining seated position.

GREENS: The GREEN group is diverse. Some of you will never need a Quick-Relief Strategy to decrease your pain. For those of you who do, it will likely be comprised of 3-4 stretches and one position to decrease your pain.

3c) SUGGESTED POSITIONS AND STRETCHES

Following are some positions and stretches to consider as you develop a Quick-Relief Strategy:

RECLINING: A position that decreases pain for many people is reclining with your back in the neutral position and a bend at the knees and hips. Most of you can achieve the neutral position in a chair that reclines and has a firm back, like a reclining chair, an executive chair, or a rocker with your feet on a stool or ottoman. You can also recline flat on a firm bed or firm couch with pillows under your knees. You can also recline on your couch or bed with a wedge behind your trunk that completely supports your trunk from hips to head. Make sure you are your neutral or most pain free position. When you use a wedge, make sure that you bend at your hips and not in your back.

FLOOR CLOCK: Another position that decreases pain for many people is the floor clock, which is also described in the exercise program in Chapter 7. Lie on your back with your hips and knees bent, either with your feet on the floor or with your legs over a chair. How close the chair is to your hips depends on your pain and where you need the chair to be to put your back in the neutral or most pain-free position. Likewise, use a chair that is the right height to get your back in the neutral or most pain-free position. Your arms will probably be most comfortable at your sides with your hands resting on your abdomen. The first time try this for just 5 minutes to see if any other part of your body is unhappy in this position. If there are no problems, slowly build up to being able to hold the position for 45 minutes.

POSITIONAL TRACTION: Positional Traction can decrease pain that is on one side of the back or down one leg. It uses the same principle as described in Pattern VI, bending away from and rotating towards the painful side to decrease your pain. The idea is to lie in a position that opens up the side of the back that is painful. To achieve Positional Traction, lie on your side with the painful side up and with two pillows between your legs from your knees to your feet. If your waist is smaller than your hips, add a small pillow under your side. Note how much pain you have. Slowly start to rotate your upper body backward about ½ inch at a time while keeping your lower body still, or start by keeping your upper body still and slowly rotating your hips forward. For most people the pain decreases after you move a little. Stop in the position where the pain is absent or you are in the least painful position. When you keep moving past the least painful position the pain will start to increase. Hold in the least painful position for several minutes, as tolerated. If your pain does not decrease, stop the activity and move out of the position. Hold off on this position until your PT recommends trying it again. In the full positional traction position you do not use pillows; the upper body is completely rolled back and the lower body, hips, and pelvis are completely rolled forward, to open up the low back. However, this full position is too much initially for most people.

HALF KNEELING: For those of you who have back pain when you arch your back, stretching the front of the thigh while in the half kneeling position frequently provides relief. This is most helpful if the back can be positioned in a neutral position during the stretch. See instructions for hip extension stretch in half kneeling position in Chapter 7. Review the best technique with your physical therapist.

SEATED LOW BACK STRETCH: For those of you who can decrease your pain by slightly or fully flattening your back, the seated low back stretch forward, can provide some relief. See instructions for seated low back stretch in chapter 7. Review the best technique with your physical therapist.

INSTRUCTIONS FOR CHART 3c. As you determine positions that decrease your pain write them down in the Chart 3c. Try to find positions that you can easily assume at home, work and/or school. As you determine stretches that decrease your pain write them down in the Chart 3c.

Chart 3c Quick Relief Strategy

Quick-Relief Positions	Instruction Notes

Quick-Relief Stretches	Instruction Notes

PAIN AS A GUIDE FOR YOUR PROGRESS

Pain as your roadmap

The information you learn in your Protective Program is essential for the overall success of both your Protective Program and your Corrective Program. It is very important to grasp the significance of this point: pain is the best road map you have for getting you out of the trouble you are in. Listen closely to your pain.

It is easy to temporarily decrease your pain. It is much more challenging to effectively address your limitations and regain the mechanics to perform your full range of activities without pain. Pay attention to the details; pay attention to your pain.

Plan ahead

As you use your Protective Program, remember to think beyond the lists. Be careful to keep your back in your neutral or most pain-free position as you move through your day. Plan ahead, consider your tolerance for activities and outings. If driving long distances is painful for you, plan to stop to get out and walk around. If the activity requires much standing and if standing is painful for you, possibly arrive late and leave early. Check to see if where you are going has a place where you can pursue your best positions. In your home, get creative to find ways to help your back into its best position without having to work to keep it there; for example, if flattening your back decreases your pain, use a stool to put your feet up when you sit in order to flatten your back. This is a better position of rest than having to constantly contract your abdominal muscles to flatten your back.

Relationship between your Protective and Corrective Programs

Your pain is presently giving you feedback, which provides you with a good deal of information. This is an opportunity to learn about your back and how to manage it. If you lose this learning opportunity, your back will likely provide you with another opportunity to learn by repeating this painful condition.

You might experience a significant decrease in pain when you start your Protective Program, before you start your Corrective Program. Be aware that by protecting your back and decreasing your pain, you are essentially turning off your warning system while not yet addressing the underlying mechanical problems that cause the pain.

No matter how good you feel, make sure you follow through with your Corrective Program to address your underlying problems.

Your Corrective Program

INTRODUCTION

YOUR exercise plan in the System Limitations Approach to Pain is called your Corrective Program. This is your opportunity to address specific mechanical limitations in your body that force your back into poor positions or force your back to perform activities it was not designed to do on a regular basis.

The exercise program is customized to your body, designed to address your specific mechanical limitations in positions that protect your back and do not increase your pain. To effectively improve your mechanics in a way that does not further aggravate your back and that carries over to your life's activities, requires consideration of many factors while you develop each exercise. This chapter includes a list of principles to use while you build each exercise and develop the program as a whole.

Research reveals that exercise is helpful in the prevention of back pain. However, once you have back pain, exercise has been found to be only slightly helpful. Most exercise programs are generalized programs adapted to you in broad terms. I believe the effectiveness of exercise for the treatment of back pain will significantly increase with this approach since your body is measured to find out *specifically* which exercises you need, tailoring your exercise program to your pain, your limitations, and your activities.

Before explaining the building blocks for your Corrective Program, it's important to know how to minimize pain and problems that could inadvertently be aggravated as you begin your exercises.

GUIDELINES TO MINIMIZE PAIN DURING YOUR CORRECTIVE PROGRAM

Pain has a significant role in the development of your Corrective Program. You want to use the feedback your pain provides to help develop your program. Since these exercises directly address the mechanical limitations that cause your back problems a slight change in technique could elicit the same force that caused your back pain to begin with. To minimize the number of problems that arise, follow the principles in this chapter to develop each exercise. As problems will arise, following are some strategies to address those problems.

HAVE A QUICK-RELIEF STRATEGY

Be sure to have a Quick-Relief Strategy prior to starting your Corrective Program. You develop a Quick-Relief Strategy as part of your Protective Program. This way if you start an exercise that turns out to aggravate your back or if you overdo an exercise (which happens to everyone), you are not stuck at home with increased pain; you have something you can do on your own to decrease your pain.

WE'RE FINE AS IS, LEAVE US ALONE

During treatment you will start to have new pains. It might be hard to imagine, but despite your back pain, part of your body is happy in its present physical state. It could be that part of your body is on vacation and not interested in coming back to work. When you start working to improve your mechanics, those areas speak up with all sorts of new sensations. This sensation will be in a different location than the original pain, or, if in the same location, it will be a different quality. You might experience it as the type of soreness you would expect with a new athletic event, rather than as a pain that feels threatening.

Report all these new sensations to your PT, although, most of the new sensations resolve by themselves. Work with your PT on any that do not resolve.

RED FLAGS—STOP!

Look for red flags; issues that you need to address immediately. In the case of all red flags, stop the program and call your physician.

- **Loss of bowel and bladder control:** Call your physician and go to the hospital immediately.
- **Diabetes out of control:** Call your physician immediately.
- **Changes in blood pressure or cardiac issues that are warning signs for needing help:** Call your physician immediately.

YELLOW FLAGS—SLOW DOWN!

Yellow flags are issues you need to address, too. Call your physical therapist, modify your Corrective Program and, as needed, look at your Protective Program to pursue the positions that decrease your pain.

- **Decreased strength:** Call your physical therapist or physician immediately.
- **Increase in intensity of original pain:** As a rule, once you develop your Corrective Program

the exercises should not increase the original pain. When you are learning the techniques for new exercises you might experience increased pain. There are some normal ups and downs in your pain. Call your PT to help you sort out whether your increased pain is typical and not alarming or a problem that requires attention.

- **New back or leg pain:** Call your PT and discuss what is happening; modify your exercise program accordingly.
- **New pain/sensation with irritating or aggravating quality:** Stop the exercises and call your PT.
- **New pain/sensation that persists or gets worse**: This is something to pay attention to. Call your PT and inform them of what you are experiencing. The natural course is that old pain and new pain will come and go. Some of the new pain is just an area that you are waking up to get it back to work and that area is protesting; most of that sensation just resolves itself while you keep progressing forward. You want to take care of everything. You don't want to lose your forward progress chasing around new sensations that will resolve by themselves. How long you and your PT should wait to address it depends on the nature and severity of the sensation. I usually address a pain of higher intensity in a couple days if it does not resolve itself. I usually address a pain of lower intensity within two weeks if it does not resolve itself.
- **Problems with balance:** With increased flexibility you might feel looser and experience a feeling of decreased balance. This is particularly important to note if you already have a balance problem. Take precautions to minimize the risk of a fall. Tell your PT about this.
- **New sensation over the top of the shoulder or outside of the upper arm:** It might increase when raising your arm up in front, out to the side, or behind you. Stop all arm exercises that cause sensation in your shoulder. Inform your PT.
- **New sensation on the outside of the hip:** This is pain that increases when you move your leg out to the side or when lying on your side. Stop any exercises which involves moving your leg out and increases sensation on the outside of your hip. Inform your PT.

READ YOUR BODY'S CUES

Refer back to the section about the roles of pain in Chapter 3 to help you understand what cues your body gives you. You should have less pain after you exercise than you had before. Ideally your pain should diminish in intensity or size as a result of your exercise program. If your pain was a 3/10 when you started, it is okay if you are a 3/10 after the exercise—but it is not okay if your pain increases to a 4/10. If the intensity stays the same but is now somewhere else, this means the exercise decreased one pain and increased another; discuss this with your PT to make adjustments in your exercise.

If your pain increases right after the exercises or an hour later, it is probably caused by one of the exercises, not the whole program. The problem exercise is usually the one that you do not like. If you do not know which exercise increases your pain, try to figure it out by noting how you feel just before and after each exercise. Work on this with your PT. Once you identify the exercise that increases your pain, review the technique with your PT. If your technique is right, something needs to be changed about the exercise, or the exercise needs to be changed altogether.

Don't push developing your Corrective Program too fast. When you work slowly and methodically to develop your program, starting small and adding just a few new exercises at a time, it is much easier to read your body's cues than if you do too much too fast. Your PT will help you interpret your body's cues as you move carefully through all of these steps.

Your goal is to have an exercise program to that does not increase your pain as you address your mechanical limitations.

LIST OF ALL THE PRINCIPLES OF YOUR CORRECTIVE PROGRAM

Here are fifteen important principles of your Corrective Program. You and your PT will apply these principles to different phases of your program's development.

The following list includes all the principles that apply to your Corrective Program. Keep reading! This chapter provides explanations and details for all these principles.

PRINCIPLES TO DEVELOP EACH EXERCISE:

1. Build your exercise program from your list of mechanical limitations.
2. Address one mechanical limitation at a time.
3. Exercise in your most pain-free functional positions.
4. When possible, choose exercise positions that mimic life activities.
5. STOP! Achieve your neutral back position before proceeding.
6. The exercise technique is important to your outcome.
7. Use pain as your guide.

PRINCIPLES TO GUIDE YOUR ENTIRE INITIAL PROGRAM

8. Start small and add.
9. Exercise daily.
10. Work toward a trial of independent management.

PRINCIPLES FOR PROGRESSING YOUR CORRECTIVE PROGRAM

11. Return to your PT for re-evaluation.
12. Your PT re-measures you as you can tolerate.
13. Your new measurements help your PT adjust your program.
14. Learn your final Corrective Program.

15. Discuss lifetime exercise possibilities.

DEVELOPING YOUR INITIAL
CORRECTIVE PROGRAM

Following are the first ten principles in more detail, followed by techniques to address the different mechanical limitations.

PRINCIPLES #1-7 TO DEVELOP EACH EXERCISE

Principle #1: Build your exercise program from your list of mechanical limitations. You each have your own set of mechanical limitations and your own ways of compensating for them, so your exercise program is unique to you. As you try each exercise and adapt each one to your needs, you build a program that is subtly different than any other person's program. Those subtle differences have a significant impact on the success of your program. This is an important reason to develop this program with a physical therapist who can customize it for you.

Principle #2: Address one mechanical limitation at a time. Each exercise focuses on just one mechanical limitation at a time rather than stretching or strengthening a number of areas of your body at the same time. Your PT helps you focus your attention where it's needed for each exercise.

Principle #3: Exercise in your most pain-free functional position. Pick the best functional position for the exercise, the one that is least likely to aggravate your back pain, standing, sitting, or lying down. You and your PT use your knowledge of which activities and which specific back positions increase your pain and which decrease your pain. Your PT might need to modify the functional positions for some exercises so that they work for you.

Principle #4: When possible, choose exercise positions that mimic life activities. Exercise positions should be designed for optimal carry-over to daily activities. The position of the body—specifically the joint above and the joint below the area being stretched or strengthened—should mimic how the body ideally uses the area during daily life, whenever it is possible.

Principle #5: Stop! Achieve your neutral back position before proceeding. This is a primary principle that you need to take into account as you develop each exercise. After you select the limitation to address and the position to exercise in, move your back into the neutral position. Contract your abdominals to hold your back in that position. Then proceed with the exercise maintaining the neutral position throughout the exercise. Retraining your back to stay in neutral is a big part of the improvement in mechanics you are working to achieve.

If you cannot achieve a neutral position or if it is painful, start with your most pain-free position. As you make progress and your neutral position is increasingly pain-free, you will work toward using your neutral position for most exercises.

Principle #6: The exercise technique is critical to your outcome. Technique means how gentle or hard you stretch, how long you hold the exercise, etc. A segment discussing exercise technique for each of the Big Four Mechanics follows this section.

Principle #7: Use pain as your guide. Pain guides you in the development of your exercise program by giving feedback during and after each exercise. Refer to the section on the Roles of Pain in Chapter 3 and the section in this chapter on Guidelines to Minimize Pain during Your Corrective Program.

Developing the exercises using all the principles comes very easily for some of you. For others it might take 30 minutes or more to develop one exercise that does not increase your pain and meets some of the principles.

PRINCIPLES #8-10 TO GUIDE YOUR ENTIRE INITIAL PROGRAM

Principle #8: Start small and add. Your PT starts with three exercises that most easily integrate the principles above. You go home, work on the exercises, and see how your body responds to them. During each session with your PT report how the exercises went at home and review the techniques. When you add just three exercises at a time, if your symptoms increase after you exercise it is easier to figure out which exercise is the problem.

The reason for starting small and adding is to easily identify and address problems with your exercise program. There are many reasons that you could have increased pain while you are building your exercise program. If a technique is accidentally altered, if you push too fast, or if the exercise is not the right one for you at this time, you can aggravate your back. Working methodically from the beginning, you minimize the risk of aggravating your back; and when you do, you can more easily find the problem. So starting small and adding is the most efficient means to build a solid program that your back tolerates. Working methodically helps reduce the frequency and severity of errors.

Principle #9: Exercise daily. What you do seven days a week has the greatest impact on your body. Therefore your exercise program is designed for you to perform at home, so you can do it seven days a week instead of three.

Principle #10: Work toward a trial of independent management. The signs that you are ready for a trial of independent management include the following: 1) You have an effective Protective

Program you use to independently decrease your pain; 2) You have a Corrective Program with exercises that address as many mechanical limitations as you can at the time with proper technique; and 3) You have no other physical therapy treatment needs. When you achieve all these goals and your PT feels it is appropriate, you can go on a trial of independent management—meaning that rather than going to see your PT each week, you work independently at home on your Protective and Corrective Programs.

In my practice I send patients out several times during the development of their programs for a trial period of independent management.

The time frame for a trial of independent management varies. It can be two weeks if you are in the RED or YELLOW group and need help managing your issues. It can be four, six, or eight weeks if you are doing well with your Protective and Corrective Programs. If you are in the GREEN group and are managing well on your own, your trial of independent management can be as long as twelve weeks. Any of you might need to return for physical therapy sessions sooner for a number of reasons. For example: to help you manage your pain, to adjust your home exercise program, or for some direct hands-on treatment by your PT. If you have questions or are having pain or problems, just call and make an appointment earlier than planned.

SPECIFIC TECHNIQUES TO ADDRESS MECHANICAL LIMITATIONS

Following are techniques for addressing each type of mechanical limitation. Back patients and physical therapists will benefit from research on exercise technique, focusing on the most effective exercise to address different mechanical limitations, different body types and how the improvement can best carry over to daily life. Meanwhile I have found the following techniques demonstrate the most improvement as shown by re-measurements.

Increase your range of motion: gentle stretching

There are many reasons to stretch. In this program the purpose is to increase your range of motion so as to move the way you were designed to move. Each exercise is designed to increase the range of motion needed in a particular part of your body, doing so while your back stays in neutral.

Re-measurements in my PT practice reveal that many traditional stretches do not effectively increase range of motion. Stretching to get a big stretch sensation typically results in minimal increase in range of motion

The stretching technique I have found most effective is to hold the stretch right at the point where you feel the first sensation. The time to hold a stretch depends on the tissue requiring increased motion. Most stretches are for ten to thirty seconds. If the position is comfortable and you can rest during the stretch, it can be held for three to five minutes. However, power muscles like those down the back of the leg, the bottom muscles, the thigh muscles, and the calf muscles demonstrate the most improvement when the stretch is held at the sign of the first sensation for two seconds or less. It seems that the muscles that are easiest to strengthen are the most difficult to stretch and the muscles that are easiest to stretch are the most difficult to strengthen.

In the most effective stretches the sensation subsides while you hold the stretch; it is also okay if the sensation stays the same. However an *increase* in the stretch sensation during the hold indicates that something is uncomfortable and you need to stop the stretch. In that case correct your position and try that stretch again. If you get the same results, stop that specific stretch for that session and try it during the next session. If it is still a problem, put that exercise on hold and ask your physical therapist to review it with you. You might need to change either your technique or the entire exercise.

Improve your motor control: start stabilization exercises

While your back does not need to be completely still in all of life's activities, most of you either use your back much more than it was designed to move or have your back in a poor position during activity. In the System Limitations Approach to back pain, the goal for motor control is to be able to control your back in the neutral position while you perform an activity with your arms and legs, or position yourself at rest. Trunk stabilization exercises, if done correctly, teach your body that skill.

Motor control starts in your brain. If the movement started in the leg rather than the brain, people with spinal cord injuries would be able to move their legs. Your brain is the software for motor control; it controls your back position, which part of your body moves, which part is still, and which muscles do the job.

I believe in very strict training for trunk stabilization. If you are unable to achieve neutral or if neutral is painful, you might need to start with positioning your back in the most pain-free position. As you make progress, neutral generally becomes your most comfortable and pain-free position.

The problem with many "trunk stabilization" or "core stabilization" exercises advertised today is that most people with back pain do not have the range of motion or strength to perform the exercise properly in a manner that keeps the back stable in the neutral position. Repetitively moving your back during the exercise trains your back to continue to move during daily activity rather than training your brain to control your back in the neutral position. No matter what the exercise is called, if your back is moving throughout the exercise, in my opinion it is not a back stabilization exercise.

In all trunk stabilization exercises, start by moving your back into the neutral position and concentrate on keeping it there. Set up a way to monitor whether your back stays in the correct position. I do not like any device that has something like a bag of air across your back to measure pressure, because your back could shift and the pressure stays the same. Once you determine a way to effectively ensure that your back stays still in the neutral or most pain-free position, start the exercise. If your back moves out of the neutral or most pain-free position, stop the exercise. Re-position and start again. Work up to being able to perform the exercise with your back in neutral for two minutes.

If you have significant back pain and significant mechanical limitations, you have been moving your back to help accomplish most of your activity for a long time. You might feel that the motor control exercises are impossible because you cannot even start to pick up a leg without your back moving to help. Your starting point for the exercise might have to be just thinking about moving your leg or just lifting a slight bit of weight off the leg. Any more attempt to lift your leg than that and your back will move too. If you let your back move, you are just training your body to continue to use your back to move your legs during activity. You want the activity to come from the hips, and so this is a critical exercise in accomplishing your goal of stopping your back from doing more than it was designed for. If you are strict with your exercise and do not let your back move, eventually you will be able to lift a leg without moving your back. For those who use their back frequently this can take months to accomplish.

For many reasons I believe the best exercise to start with is the hook-lying position; see Chapter 7 for instructions in hook-lying stabilization exercises. In this position it is easy to achieve the neutral back position, gravity does not interfere with the exercise, and the floor contact provides feedback about the position of your back. Once you can perform the hook-lying stabilization exercise and you can hold your back still and lift your leg, you can try other exercise positions for motor control. For any new exercise you need to have enough range of motion to be able to perform the exercise without causing your back to move.

With your PT's help, you can add other stabilization exercises that relate to your life activities. For example, if you row a boat you can use an exercise that recreates your rowing position and arm motions.

Once you have the right technique for the stabilization exercise, performing it repetitively is the key to learning. Just as in any sporting activity, repetitively performing a skill helps you learn it to the point that it becomes an automatic activity.

Remember: Make sure that for any trunk stabilization exercises, you move your back into its neutral position, and that you have the range of motion and strength to allow your back to stay in the neutral position while performing the exercise.

Improve your postural alignment: re-educate your body

When you start to improve your range of motion, motor control, and strength, your body does not necessarily automatically know what to do with these improvements. Your next step in physical therapy is to slowly and repetitively teach your body what your new postural alignment should be with your improved mechanics. What you need for your posture is individual and unique to you. It is important that your physical therapist helps you learn what you need to do to correct your posture.

The most important thing to remember is that *you cannot completely correct your posture right away.* Many of you moved into your present poor alignment to avoid a problem in your body. Forcing your body back into a more upright alignment before your mechanics can support it can cause problems and pain. As you gradually regain the range of motion, motor control, and strength you need for better posture, you will be able to move into better postural alignment.

The best technique I have found to improve posture is with small steps from the bottom up. For example, start by shifting your hips back over the top of your ankle joints or tilting your bottom under to decrease the arch in your back. Then make small adjustments to your upper body. Try a number of different cues to get your upper body to a better postural position. For example, imagine there is a rope attached to the top of your head and the rope lifts you up bringing your trunk into better alignment, or take a deep breath to open up your chest and move your shoulders back; when you relax your breath try to maintain the same chest position with shoulders back.

Once you and your PT find the right cues to achieve your best current upright position, relax your body underneath and hold this position. Depending on your mechanical issues, hold it anywhere from five seconds to a couple of minutes. During that time pay close attention to what this position feels like. Let it sink in that this is the new alignment you want to achieve. Work on your postural changes several times throughout the day, and slowly increase the time, repetition and the number of improvements.

Increase your strength: address areas of weakness

The reason to strengthen in this program is to address the specific limitations in your strength that impact your back.

Your physical therapist will select your strengthening exercises based on your list of mechanical limitations. If you have not tolerated a manual muscle test but are ready to start some strengthening, your posture will usually indicate which muscles to concentrate on. For many it is the abdominals, the upper back muscles, and the leg muscles, including the gluteal muscles over the bottom. Your physical therapist will choose your exercise positions based on all the principles listed in the beginning of this chapter.

Once you know the limitation to address and the position for a particular exercise, you can start the exercise. Position your back in neutral, make sure you contract your abdominals to stabilize your trunk and begin focusing your movement on the muscle you want to strengthen. Stay within your joints' current range of motion and your muscles' ability to perform the exercise; otherwise you might pull your back out of its neutral position to help perform the exercise.

You want to strengthen the muscle in the manner in which it functions. Some muscles are designed to provide power, and some are designed to provide stability to your body. The power muscles contract forcefully for a short duration, and the stabilizers contract at a low level over a long period of time. For example, the biceps muscle in the arm happily produces the power to lift an object but is very unhappy about having to hold the contraction over a long period of time. You might experience this when you lift an object; initially your arms are fine, but when you have to hold it longer (for example, while waiting for someone to open the door), your arms might start to shake a little. In contrast, the muscles in your upper back between your shoulder blades will contract at a low level for a long period of time while you work at a computer. Difficulty holding yourself up at the computer could suggest limited strength in the postural stability muscles in your upper back. Keep in mind that some muscles might have a variety of jobs.

PROGRESSING YOUR CORRECTIVE PROGRAM

PRINCIPLES #11-15

This section gives you a general idea of what to expect as you progress your program. You need to continually customize your program to your unique body and its changing needs. Your physical therapist will work with you on the specific details of how to progress your exercises, including how to alter stretches to achieve different angles of stretch and how to best increase weights.

Principles #11-13 are discussed in Chapter 4 about evaluations. I am repeating some of that information here so it is available at hand when you are working on each part.

Principle #11: Return to your PT for re-evaluation. A re-evaluation compares your present status with your initial status, focusing on the progress you've made with your activity level, your mechanics, and your pain. The re-evaluation also looks at how you are doing overall with your program and any problems you are having in managing your body. You might not have re-measurements at every re-evaluation; this depends on your pain, how easily your pain is aggravated, and how long it has been since your last re-measurement. When you do not have re-measurements, a detailed, objective and measurable description of your pain gives you important information about your progress.

Principle #12: Your PT re-measures you as much as you can tolerate. Re-measurements help your PT evaluate how effective your exercises are at improving your mechanics. For most of you, the first re-measurements of your limitations will be 9-12 weeks after you complete the development of your initial exercise program. Further re-measurements will ideally be scheduled at 12-week intervals. You need time for the exercises to be effective, yet longer than 12 weeks is too long to do an exercise that is not working. For some in the RED group repeated range of motion measurements might be too aggravating and therefore counterproductive. You might wait much longer than 12 weeks to have re-measurements.

Principle #13: Your new measurements help your PT adjust your program. Re-measurements provide data about how effectively your exercises are addressing your mechanical limitations. If your re-measurements demonstrate progress, you will continue your exercises until you reach your goals. If your re-measurements do not demonstrate progress, your PT will look at your exercise technique and at how often you do the exercises to see if there are any problems with your present program. S/he might make adjustments in the exercises or change the exercise altogether.

Continue with intervals of re-measurements until you and your physical therapist think you have maximized the development of your program and have progressed as far as you can with your mechanics. Many of you have had mechanical limitations for years, even decades, and you will be able to continue making progress for years if you stick with your Corrective Program. If you have residual limitations, you might need to continue with your program to maintain your status while you await new ideas or new research to address your residual limitations.

Principle #14: Learn your final Corrective Program. When you improve your mechanics as much as you can, you need to work with your PT to design your final Corrective Program. Which exercises are important for you to continue in order to maintain your improved mechanics? Which exercises need to be done the most frequently? Everyone should exercise at least three times a week. Your Corrective Program is designed for your individual needs and should be a part of your ongoing exercise program

Principle #15: Discuss lifetime exercise possibilities. Before you part ways with your physical therapist, think together about any physical activity that you wish to start or resume. Discuss lifetime exercise interests of yours, such as, walking, home exercise video, bicycling, weight training, yoga, pilates, swimming, skiing, tennis, etc. Your body and mind benefit from exercise. For the exercises you are interested in, discuss what aspects are safe for you and what aspects are risky for you.

FINISHING WITH YOUR PHYSICAL THERAPIST

CURRENT REGULATIONS

Current PT regulations require that the physical therapist formally discharge the patient from therapy. The typical routine is that the patient sees the PT for a number of consecutive weeks and then is discharged when s/he begins independent work. Unlike other medical practitioners who treat patients for years working from the same medical chart, the PT is required to discharge the patient. The chart is not kept open, and if the patient returns the PT needs to perform a whole new evaluation and start a new chart.

For many of you whose pain is caused by mechanical limitations, these mechanical limitations are usually still present as your independent work begins. If you return to your PT for more help, your underlying problem remains the same. Yet the present structure requires a whole new evaluation, which is costly and inefficient.

WHAT IS NEEDED?

Addressing your mechanical limitations can be a long and complicated process. When your pain is caused by mechanical limitations, you would benefit from having your PT's guidance until you reach the goal of improving your mechanics. Access to your PT throughout this process can facilitate your progress, minimize recurrence, minimize the chance of progressively getting worse, and decrease the overall cost of repeated evaluations and paperwork.

I hope to see the regulations revised, to structure treatment in a way that addresses the underlying problems with greater overall efficiency and access to physical therapists as consultants over an extended time frame.

GOALS

Your goals are centered around three topics: your pain, your activity or functional level, and your mechanical limitations.

Your PT works with you on your goals at the time of your evaluation. If you are in the RED or YELLOW group your goals will be modified over time as your PT gets to know you better. Some of you will have goals of becoming 100 percent pain-free and returning to all activities. Some of you will have goals of being able to take care of yourself while engaging in only light activities and accepting that there will still be some pain. These goals are based on your history, how long you've had pain, how intense it has been, the extent of your mechanical limitations, and the changes in your back seen on films such as MRI.

First and foremost, try your best with your program. Undoubtedly there will be goals you do not meet. Ideal alignment and full range of motion, strength, and motor control are used as a means for measurement and a direction to move toward, but most of us never had that and will never achieve that. Customize your goals and achievements. The mechanics you improve and the pain you decrease will focus on the health of your body and on achieving activities you need and are interested in. Keep your focus on you. Do your best to get as far as you can to take care of your body.

FINISHING SCENARIOS

There are as many scenarios for finishing with the PT as there are people who have back pain. You finish with your PT when you have met all of your goals. You might also finish with your PT if you have not met all your goals but have exhausted the avenues available trying to meet those goals.

Remember, it is not enough to only meet your pain goal, or even both your pain goal and your activity goals. You have a better chance of avoiding recurrence of your pain if you also achieve the goals for your mechanical limitations.

When your efforts do not decrease your pain, your PT will work with you to try and figure out if, a) you have achieved your best possible mechanics, b) you are on the right track but need more time or need to adjust the program, c) you need an opinion from another PT. (No one person knows everything and another physical therapy opinion should be okay with your present PT), d) your pain possibly stems from another source, in which case you need to follow up with your doctor. This is a time when having a detailed, objective, measurable description of your pain from the beginning helps immensely. If you tracked your progress closely you see over time what helped and what did not. This information helps you in the end if you have unresolved issues; this is a significant reason for having the detailed description to begin with.

People will make different choices. Some of you will decide to keep your activities to a level that keeps you pain-free. Some of you will always push yourselves, never stopping until something like pain stops you. Some of you will make a choice in between, to push only at certain times. The choice is yours. My mother used to go all out when the grandchildren visited. Many times she would pay for that for weeks, but she was content with her decision.

When you have mechanical limitations that do not improve and you have exhausted the avenues of known treatment, make sure you know which limitations you are struggling with. Then keep your eye out for new research offering ideas about those specific mechanical limitations.

When you finish with your PT you should have:

- a final Corrective Program
- a final Protective Program
- a Quick-Relief Strategy for each of the pains you have
- plans for life exercise/activity programs
- knowledge of the mechanical limitations that you have not met
- understanding of issues not covered by this approach, for which you have either received treatment or need treatment.

In any of the scenarios above, remember that even after you finish with your PT, if you start to have new symptoms or the return of symptoms you should call your PT or your MD.

MOTIVATION TO CONTINUE: FEELINGS OF SUCCESS

Addressing your mechanical limitations is a long-term process. You need to know where to look for feelings of success to keep yourself motivated. You can feel successful as you learn what you need to do, follow through with your program, and realize the progress you are making.

CONTROL

Control over your pain contributes significantly to feelings of success. Most of you gain a sense of control over your pain when you understand your mechanical limitations and how they affect your body. You gain control when you have your Protective Program and when you have your Quick-Relief Strategy to decrease pain on your own. Finally, you have a feeling of control when you develop your Corrective Program.

The ancient Chinese philosopher Lau Tzu famously said, "Give a man a fish and you feed him for a day. Teach a man to fish and you feed him for a lifetime." Just like learning how to fish, in the System Limitations Approach to Pain, your feeling of success comes from learning to control your pain on your own instead of having to depend on someone else.

THE ROLES OF PAIN

Review the roles of pain in Chapter 2 to better understand your pain so that you can use the signals your pain is giving you to help you feel successful and subsequently stay motivated to continue with your program.

PERFORM YOUR EXERCISE PROGRAM

Since improving your mechanics is a long process, your daily feeling of success needs to come from taking the step each day to do your exercises.

YOUR MEASURABLE IMPROVEMENTS IN BOTH ACTIVITIES AND MECHANICS

You worked hard to achieve a detailed, measurable and objective description of your experience with pain in the first step of your Protective Program. For many of you, reading the initial description of your pain and activity helps you clearly see your success. For most people, I find reading the initial description to be the single most effective source of motivation.

Likewise, your PT took very specific baseline measurements of your mechanics to identify the cause of your pain and to track the effectiveness of your exercises. After your pain is gone measurable improvements continue in your mechanics as you continue your exercises. Re-measurements of your mechanics can help keep you motivated to continue with your exercise program for two reasons: 1) You know you have to face re-measurements, so you do your exercises to improve the next set of data; and 2) When you see measurable progress you feel successful and want to continue your program.

BUILD CONFIDENCE IN YOUR BODY

Experiencing a decrease in pain and seeing improvement in your measurements are nice; however, there is another benefit that you will hopefully experience—a new confidence in your body. The pain subsides, you continue your Corrective Program, and, increasingly, you realize you can count on your body. You feel like you can tackle a greater range of activities for a longer time without an immediate pain response from your body. This is a wonderful feeling of success.

CHAPTER 7

Exercise Instruction
List of Exercises, Instructions, and Pictures

INTRODUCTION

THE following are instructions for exercises that I commonly use. They are examples of how to apply the principles to the exercises. I also include them here in case you and your PT want to consider some of these exercises for your program.

The exercises here are designed to improve range of motion, motor control, and strength. Posture exercises are not included. The exercises to correct your posture are unique to you, and your PT will decide how you can best achieve the correction you need. The instructions include techniques that have proven most effective in my practice. Ultimately research will identify which exercises are the most effective.

Your PT will select exercises to address your limitations. S/he should decide the specifics of each exercise; for example, how you will achieve neutral or your most pain free position, how long you tolerate holding each exercise, how many repetitions, how long you need to rest between each repetition, etc.

When an exercise description recommends something to hold onto or lean on, make sure you use a very sturdy object that will not collapse or move away from you.

For each exercise, take the following steps:

1. Choose the best position for the exercise.
2. Adjust your position to move your back into neutral. If there is an adjustment that is commonly used to achieve neutral, that will be noted in the instructions. If the neutral

position is painful for you, move to your most pain-free position. Contract your abdominal muscles to maintain the neutral back (or most pain-free position) as you perform the exercise.

3. Isolate the movement to address one mechanical limitation at a time.
4. Follow the recommendations for duration and repetition.

When you work on developing your exercises, some exercises might increase your pain. Work with your PT to make the necessary adjustments. The goal is to develop exercises that never increase your pain, and to find some that decrease your pain.

Be cautious of the exercises that do arch your back; do not do these when arching increases your back pain. Some exercises flatten your back; do not do these when flattening your back increases your pain. Also be cautious and stop any exercise that increases sensation on the outside of your hip or over the top of your arm when that is the aim of the exercise.

Each week I learn something new. I decided to include some instructions in the book that are more up-to-date than in the DVD, and so you will see a couple of differences between the DVD and the book instructions. For example, the placement of the foot in the calf stretch (Exercise #1) is instructed to be further in front in the book than it was in the DVD instructions.

Look for further instructions specifically for range of motion (stretching), motor control (trunk stabilization), and strength exercises at the beginning of each of those sections in this chapter.

RANGE OF MOTION

GENERAL INSTRUCTIONS FOR IMPROVING RANGE OF MOTION

You will see the term "sensation" at times instead of "stretch." Stretches to increase range of motion seem to be most effective when held at the position of the first sign of a sensation and so this is emphasized at certain times by referring to first sensation instead of stretch. You might not consider what you feel a real stretch, and so the term "sensation" is more descriptive of what to watch for. For example, when working to increase range of motion in your hamstrings, calf muscles, and bottom muscles, it is most effective to move to the point where you feel your first sensation and hold the stretch at that point for two seconds or less.

Depending on the exercise, you will hold stretches anywhere from two to thirty seconds, some eventually for four or five minutes, and one for up to forty-five minutes, depending on what has been found to be most effective so far.

To progress increase the frequency and duration but do not increase the intensity.

It is ideal if the stretch sensation subsides while you hold the stretch, 1) it is a good sign that what you feel is actually a stretch and 2) in the most successful stretches the sensation subsides while they are held. It is also okay if the sensation stays the same. However an *increase* in the stretch sensation during the hold indicates that something is aggravated and you need to stop the stretch. In that case correct your position and try that stretch again. If you get the same results, stop that specific stretch for that session and try it during the next session. If it is still a problem, put that exercise on hold and ask your physical therapist to review it with you. You might need to change either your technique or the entire exercise.

Exercise (1) Calf Stretch in Standing Position

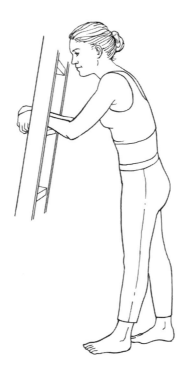

Fig. 7-1

Position: Find a sturdy object such as a counter or dresser to lean your hands on. Stand with the weight of your upper body on your hands, forearms or trunk.

Neutral Back: To achieve a neutral back position, you might need to bend forward from your hip to decrease the arch in your back. Contract your abdominals to maintain the neutral back throughout the exercise.

Isolate the Movement: The stretch is aimed at your upper calf. Place the leg to stretch on the ground about five inches in front of the other foot. Keeping the heel on the ground and the knee straight, slide the foot back until you feel the first stretch/sensation in your calf muscle; see Figure 7-1. Do not let the arch in your foot drop as you slide your foot back. Relax the stretch by slightly bending the knee. Straighten the knee for the next stretch and slightly bend the knee to relax the stretch.

Duration and Repetition: Hold the stretch for two seconds. Then slightly bend your knee to relax the stretch. Repeat 15 times.

Exercise (2) Hamstring Stretch in Standing Position

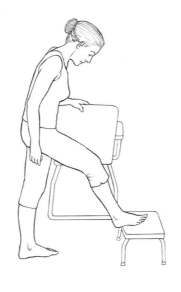

Fig. 7-2

Position: Stand with both hands on a sturdy object. (For the illustration, one object was removed so that you can see the subject.) Place one foot on a stool with the hip and knee bent.

Neutral Back: To achieve a neutral back, most of you will need to lean forward from your hip to decrease the arch in your back. Contract your abdominals to maintain the neutral back position throughout the exercise.

Isolate the Movement: The stretch is aimed at the back of the thigh of the leg on the stool. Straighten the knee until you feel the first stretch/sensation behind the thigh; see Figure 7-2. Relax the stretch by slightly bending your knee. Any shift forward of your trunk during the stretch is fine. Straighten the knee for the next stretch and slightly bend the knee to relax the stretch.

Duration and Repetition: Hold the stretch for two seconds; then bend your knee to relax. Repeat 15 times.

Exercise (3) Hip Extension Stretch in Half-Kneel Position

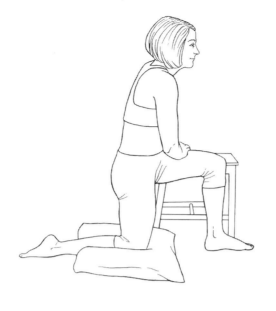

Fig. 7-3

Position: Kneel on one knee, and place the other leg out in front with knee bent so that the foot is under the knee. For balance, hold onto something sturdy with both hands. (For the illustration, one object was removed so that you can see the subject.)

Neutral Back: To achieve a neutral back position, you might need to bend forward at your hip to decrease the arch in your back. Contract your abdominals to maintain the neutral back position throughout the exercise.

Isolate the Movement: The stretch is aimed at the front of the leg that is kneeling on the ground. The stretch sensation can be felt anywhere from your hip to your knee. Tuck your bottom under until you feel the stretch in your thigh; see Figure 7-3. Relax the stretch by un-tucking your bottom. Relax by releasing your bottom muscles. Tuck your bottom under for the next stretch and then un-tuck to relax. An alternative to tucking your bottom under is to tighten your bottom muscles until you feel a stretch.

Duration and Repetition: Hold a gentle stretch for 20 seconds. Repeat three times.

Exercise (4) Hamstring Stretch in Half–Kneel Position

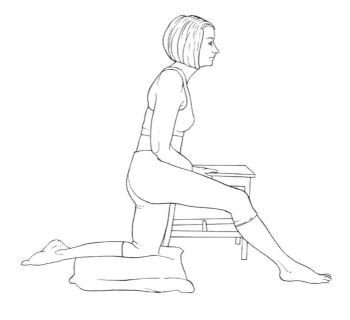

Fig. 7-4

Position: Kneel on one knee. For balance, hold onto something sturdy with both hands. (For the illustration, one object was removed so that you can see the subject.)

Neutral Back: You might need to lean forward slightly from the hip to decrease the arch in your back. Contract your abdominals to maintain the neutral back position throughout the exercise.

Isolate the Movement: The stretch is aimed at the back of the thigh of the front leg. The stretch can be felt anywhere in the back of your thigh. Slide your front leg forward, straightening your knee until you feel the first stretch/sensation in the back of your thigh; see Figure 7-4. Slightly bend your knee to relax the stretch. Straighten your knee for the next stretch and then slightly bend the knee to relax the stretch.

Duration and Repetition: Hold two seconds; slightly bend your knee to relax. Repeat 15 times.

Exercise (5) Hamstring Stretch in Long Sit Position

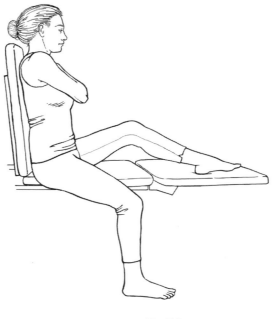

Fig. 7-5

Position: Sitting on a firm surface with your back up against a wall and one leg off the side with the foot resting on the floor. This can be done on a firm bed that is up against a wall or up against a flat head board.

Neutral Back: Prior to sitting down move your back into your neutral or most pain free back position. As you sit down have the leg on the bed bent at the knee and hip, keep your back in the neutral or most pain free position. If you can not keep your back in the neutral or most pain free position this exercise might not be for you at this.

Isolate the Movement: The stretch is aimed at the back of the thigh of the leg on the bed. Slowly straighten the knee, of the leg on the bed, until you feel the first sensation behind your thigh; see Figure 7-5. Hold that stretch 2 seconds, slightly bend your knee to relax the stretch. Straighten the knee for next stretch and slightly bend the knee to relax the stretch.

Duration and Repetition: Hold the stretch for two seconds or less, and then relax by bending your knee slightly. Repeat 15 times.

Exercise (6) Hamstring Stretch in Lying Down Position

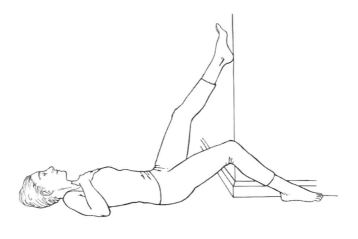

Fig. 7-6

Position: Lie on your back on the floor near a door. Position yourself so one leg can go through the door and the other leg can slide up the wall.

Neutral Back: The leg on the floor controls your back position. If that leg slides out straight, your back arches. If that leg slides too close to your body, your back flattens. The tendency in this exercise is for your back to flatten as your leg slides up the wall. You want to keep your back in neutral, and so you need to consciously maintain the neutral position and not let your back flatten when placing your leg on the wall or when sliding your leg up the wall. Contract your abdominals to maintain the neutral back position throughout the exercise.

Isolate the Movement: The stretch is aimed at the back of the thigh of the leg on the wall. Slide your leg up the wall until you feel the first stretch/sensation in the back of your thigh; see Figure 7-6. At the first sensation, hold the stretch and then bend the knee slightly to relax the stretch. Repeat straightening your knee to feel a sensation and slightly bending your knee to relax. Keep your heel still so that it does not slide up and down the wall with each repetition; the rest of your foot can move however it wants.

Duration and Repetition: Hold the stretch for two seconds or less, and then relax by bending your knee slightly. Repeat 15 times.

Exercise (7) Hip Flexion Stretch in Lying Down Position

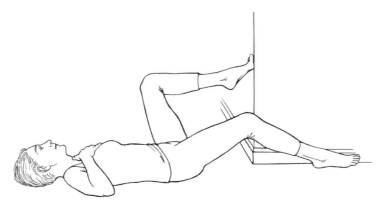

Fig. 7-7

Position: Lie on your back on the floor near a door. Position yourself so one leg can go through the door and the other leg can slide up the wall.

Neutral Back: The leg on the floor controls your back position. If that leg slides out straight, your back will arch. If that leg slides close to your body, your back will flatten. The tendency in this exercise is for your back to flatten. You want your back to maintain the neutral position and not flatten when you place your leg on the wall, when you slide your leg down the wall, and when you raise your foot up onto your toes. Contract your abdominals to maintain the neutral back position throughout the exercise.

Isolate the Movement: The stretch is aimed in the area behind the hip and anywhere throughout the bottom. Start with your leg up high on the wall, (the final position for the hamstring stretch). Slide your leg down until your foot is at or slightly below knee height. Lift your heel up off the wall so you raise up on your toes, move until you feel a stretch in your bottom; see Figure 7-7. Hold the stretch at the point of any sensation you get in the area of your bottom. Then relax your foot back down on its heel. This stretch can be difficult to feel. Repeat, rise back up on your toes until you feel a sensation, hold, and then relax. You might need to adjust how far you are from the wall to achieve the stretch or to achieve the stretch without flattening your back.

Duration and Repetition: Hold the stretch two seconds, and repeat 15 times.

Exercise (8) Hip Abduction Stretch in Lying Down Position

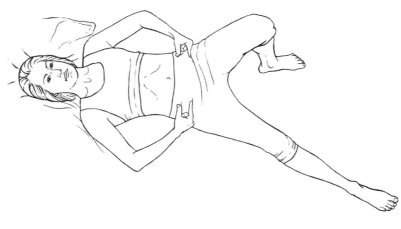

Fig. 7-8

Position: Lie on your back on the floor with one leg out straight and the other knee bent to help position your back.

Neutral Back: When you place your leg out straight, your back will arch. This time do not try to prevent the arch, because working to keep your back from arching places too much pressure on your back and pelvis. Contract your abdominal muscles to stabilize your back and prevent it from bending to the side, rotating or further arching. Place your hands on your hips to monitor for any movement in your back.

Isolate the Movement: The stretch is aimed at the inside of the leg that is straight out on the floor. Slide the leg on the floor out to the side until you feel the first sensation on the inside of your thigh; see Figure 7-8. Be sure not to move the leg too far out to the side. If you get a sensation on the outside of your hip, stop, reposition and start the exercise again. If the sensation occurs again, stop the exercise and talk to your PT.

Duration and Repetition: Hold a gentle stretch, initially for 10-20 seconds. If you do not have any increased pain with this exercise, work up to one minute.

Exercise (9) Hip Adduction Stretch in Lying Down Position

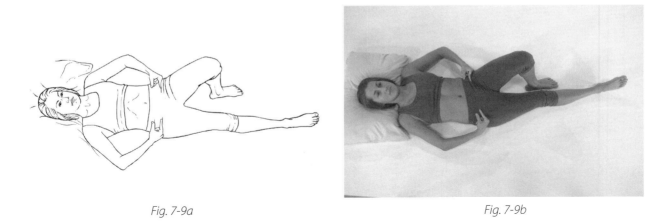

Fig. 7-9a   Fig. 7-9b

Position: Lie on your back on the floor with one knee bent to position your back and the other leg straight and out to the side. (This is the end position for the Hip Abduction stretch.)

Neutral Back: When you place one leg out straight, your back will arch. Do not try to prevent the arch, because working to keep your back from arching places too much pressure on your back and pelvis. Contract your abdominal muscles to stabilize your back and keep it bending to the side, rotating or further arching. Place your hands on your hips to monitor for any movement in your back.

Isolate the Movement: The stretch is aimed at the outside of the thigh of the leg that is straight out on the floor. Slide that leg in until you feel a sensation on the outside of your thigh. This might be just a whisper of a sensation. Hold the exercise in that position; see Figure 7-9a. If you do not feel a stretch on the outside of your hip and you move your leg past the end of your hip adduction range of motion, your back bends to the side to help move your leg; see Figure 7-9b. If that happens, reposition yourself, move your back into the neutral position again and start over. Set the leg out to the side. This time move the leg in and stop when you feel like your hands and your hips are about to move. That is the end of your hip adduction range of motion and any more movement would come from your back. You can increase your range of motion when you do not feel any stretch or sensation.

Duration and Repetition: Start with a 20-second hold. If your body is okay with this exercise and you have no increase in pain, work up to one minute.

Exercise (10) Hip Abduction Stretch in Standing Position

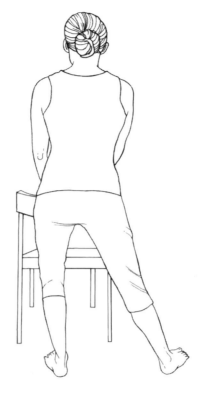

Fig. 7-10

Position: Stand with a sturdy object in front of you to hold onto, as you slide one leg out to the side as described below.

Neutral Back: To move into neutral, many of you need to decrease the arch in your back by leaning forward from the hips. The instruction for isolating movement will also help you keep your back in neutral as the back can bend to the side during this exercise. Contract your abdominals to maintain your back in the neutral position.

Isolate the Movement: The stretch is aimed at the inside of one thigh. To stretch, you will slide that leg out to the side. While you slide the leg out bend the other knee this will let your back lower down evenly, minimizing the chance that your back bends to the side; see Figure 7-10. If you get a sensation on the outside of your hip, stop, reposition and start the exercise again. If the sensation occurs again, stop the exercise and talk to your PT.

Duration and Repetition: Hold a gentle stretch for 10-20 seconds, repeat three times.

Exercise (11) Hip Adduction Stretch in Standing Position

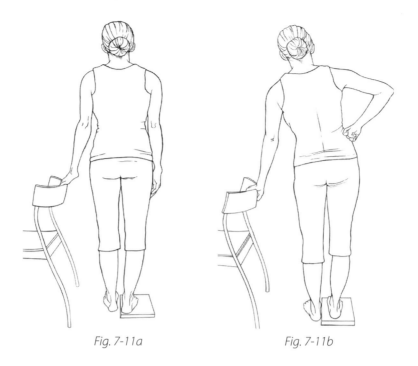

Fig. 7-11a   *Fig. 7-11b*

Position: Standing with one foot on a book and the other foot at the same height next to the foot on the book; see Figure 7-11a. The PT will determine the height of the book by your response to the stretch.

Neutral Back: Start with back in neutral position both feet at same height one on book and one off the book. The foot that is not on the book is going to be put on the floor. You need to keep your back in neutral while you do this; see Figure 7-11b.

Isolate the Movement: This is a difficult idea to describe in writing, if this exercise works for you your PT will help you learn how to move. Aim the stretch at the outside of the hip and thigh of the leg on the book. To do this the movement comes from the hip of the leg on the book. The back stays in neutral it leans to the side as the hip moves to lower the one leg down. The back joints stay in a straight neutral line rather then moving into a curved position as the back leans to the side.

As you lower the foot to the floor the back follows that leg causing the movement to come from the hip on the book. You want to feel a stretch somewhere over the outside of the thigh of the leg on the book. This is a subtle sensation.

Duration and Repetition: Hold the stretch for 15 seconds, one time. If there is no increase in symptoms try to increase to one minute, one time or 20 seconds three times.

Exercise (12) Hip Internal Rotation Stretch in Lying Down Position

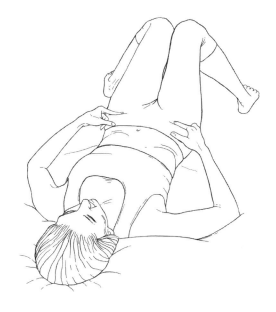

Fig. 7-12

Position: Lie on your back, hips and knees bent, with your feet and knees together.

Neutral Back: Move your back into the neutral position. Contract your abdominals to maintain the neutral position throughout the exercise.

Isolate the Movement: The stretch is aimed at your upper thighs, front inside or outside. Keeping your knees together, walk your feet out to the side until you feel a sensation somewhere over the top or sides of your upper thigh; see Figure 7-12. Do not allow your back to arch. Do not walk your feet too far. Stop, reposition, and start the exercise again if you get the sensation on the inside of your knees or at the back of your thighs. If you try again and cannot get the intended stretch, stop the exercise and talk with your PT.

Duration and Repetition: Hold the stretch at the first sign of a sensation, 10-20 seconds at first. You can build up to holding that for one minute.

Exercise (13) Hip External Rotation Stretch in Lying Down Position

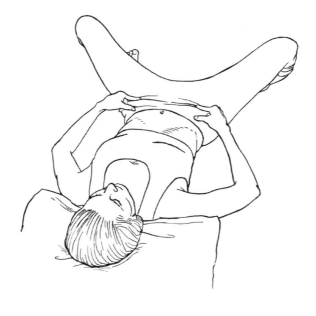

Fig. 7-13

Position: Start at the end position for the Hip Internal Rotation Stretch above, lying on the floor with your hips and knees bent, knees together, and feet out to the side.

Neutral Back: Your back should be in the neutral position prior to moving your feet out to the side. Contract your abdominals to maintain the neutral position throughout the exercise.

Isolate the Movement: The stretch is aimed at the inside of your thighs. From the starting position, lower your knees out to the side until you feel a stretch; see Figure 7-13. Make sure your back does not move. If you get a sensation on the outside of your hip, stop, reposition, and start the exercise again. If the sensation occurs again, stop the exercise and talk to your PT.

Duration and Repetition: Hold the stretch for 20 seconds, repeat three times. It is difficult to achieve a gentle stretch with this exercise.

Exercise (14) Hip Internal Rotation Stretch in Standing Position

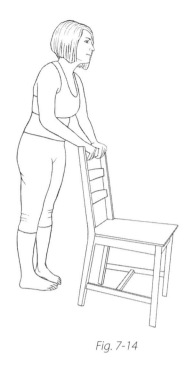

Fig. 7-14

Position: Stand and hold onto a sturdy object such as the back of a large chair, a high dresser, or counter top.

Neutral Back: You might need to bend at your hips to decrease the arch in your back and achieve a neutral position. Contract your abdominals to hold the neutral position throughout the exercise.

Isolate the Movement: The stretch is aimed at the outside of the upper thigh. Start with your feet shoulder width apart and toes slightly turned out to the side. Keeping your heels in the same position, slowly roll your legs in with the whole leg rolling in like a log, until you feel the first stretch/sensation on the outside of your thigh; see Figure 7-14. Hold the stretch at the point where you feel the first sensation

Duration and Repetition: Hold the stretch for 30 seconds to one minute.

Exercise (15) Hip External Rotation Stretch in Standing Position

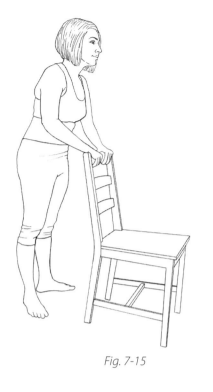

Fig. 7-15

Position: Stand and hold onto a sturdy object such as a high dresser.

Neutral Back: You might need to bend at your hips to decrease the arch in your back and achieve a neutral position. Contract your abdominals to maintain a neutral position throughout the exercise.

Isolate the Movement: The stretch is aimed at the inside of the upper thigh in the groin area. Start with your feet shoulder-width apart and toes pointing straight forward. Keeping your heels in the same position, slowly roll your legs out, rolling the whole leg like a log, until you feel a stretch on the inside of your upper thigh; see Figure 7-15. Hold the stretch at the point where you feel the first sensation. If you get a sensation on the outside of your hip, stop, reposition, and start the exercise again. If the sensation occurs again, stop the exercise and talk to your PT. You cannot do this exercise when there is a sensation on the outside of your hip; something might be getting pinched.

Duration and Repetition: Hold the stretch for 30 seconds to one minute.

Exercise (16a) Seated Low Back Stretch Forward

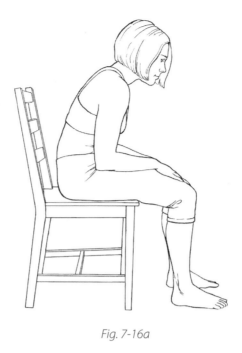

Fig. 7-16a

Position: Sit in a chair, arms resting on your thighs.

Neutral Back: This is a stretch for your back, so depending on your back you might move from a big arch to a slight arch or from neutral to flat.

Isolate the Movement: The stretch is aimed at your low back. First tilt your pelvis to flatten your back, by pulling your stomach in and tucking your bottom under; see Figure 7-16a. Stop when you feel the first stretch sensation in your low back. If you fully flatten your back and do not get a stretch sensation, start to round your back by rolling your upper body down. Stop when you feel a gentle stretch in your low back. Let your upper body weight rest on your arms. Do not bend from the hips. All the motion should come from rounding your low back. Be careful when moving back to upright to minimize the risk of catching or pinching anything in your back.

Duration and Repetition: Hold a gentle stretch for 20-30 seconds, repeat two to three times.

Exercise (16b) Seated Low Back Stretch to the Side

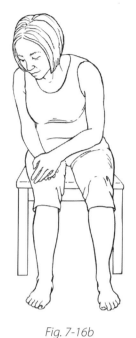

Fig. 7-16b

Position: Sit in a chair with your upper body turned towards one leg. Place both your arms on
that leg.

Neutral Back: This is a stretch for your back, so depending on your back you might move from a
big arch to a slight arch or from neutral to flattened.

Isolate the Movement: The stretch is aimed at the low back on the side you are leaning away
from. First tilt your pelvis by pulling your stomach in and tucking your bottom under. Stop
when you feel a stretch sensation in your low back. If your back is fully flattened and you
do not get a stretch sensation, start to round your back by rolling your upper body down
towards your knee. Stop when you feel the first stretch; see Figure 7-16b. Place the weight of
your upper body on your arms. Do not bend from the hips. All the motion should come from
rounding your low back. Be careful moving back to upright, to minimize the risk of catching
or pinching anything in your back.

Duration and Repetition: Hold a gentle stretch for 20-30 seconds. Repeat three times.

Exercise (17) Prone Back Stretch Forward

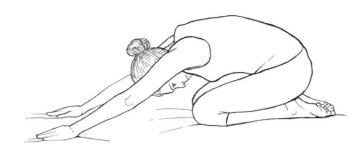

Fig. 7-17

Position: Kneel on the floor.

Neutral Back: This is a stretch for the back, so depending on your back position you might move from a big arch to a slight arch or from neutral to flat.

Isolate the Movement: The stretch is aimed the mid back and or the side of the trunk and along the outside of the shoulders. Sitting on your knees and feet and keeping your bottom on your feet, lower your upper body down toward the floor. Slide your arms out in front until you feel your first sensation. The stretch can occur anywhere from the side of your shoulder down through your middle or lower back; see Figure 7-17. Stop the exercise if you have a sensation on the top of your shoulder or arm. If this happens, reposition and try again. If it occurs again, talk with your PT. To focus the stretch on one side, leave your hips still over top of your feet and walk your upper body to one side until you feel a stretch along your side or outside of your shoulder. You can not do this exercise if you get a sensation on the side your walked your upper body towards. Same duration and repetition as when straight forward.

Duration and Repetition: Hold a gentle stretch for 20-30 seconds. Repeat three times.

Exercise (18) Pelvic Tilt

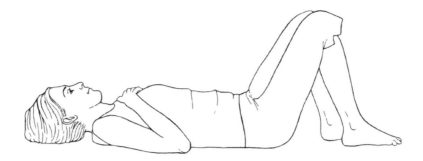

Fig. 7-18

Position: Lie on the floor with your knees and hips bent; see Figure 7-18.

Neutral Back: You will probably fall right into the neutral back position. A few people need to contract the abdominal muscles to decrease the arch and move into the neutral back position to start the exercise.

Isolate the Movement: The movement is aimed at flattening your low back onto the floor. Contract your stomach muscles to flatten your back. Move until you have a gentle stretch in your low back, and hold it there. In the beginning you might need to use your bottom muscles to help tuck your bottom under. Do not push from your feet. Gradually work on using only your stomach muscles to flatten your back.

Duration and Repetition: Hold the stretch for 20 seconds. Repeat three times. To strengthen your muscles, hold it for two seconds and repeat ten times. To increase control, contract in three steps to move the back to a flattened position and then relax in three steps returning to the neutral position.

Exercise (19) Hip Extension Stretch in Lying Down Position

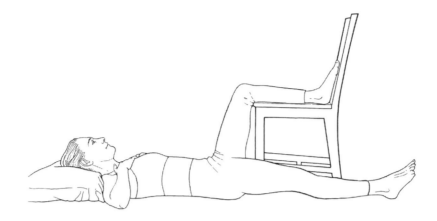

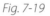
Fig. 7-19

This exercise is for you if you are working on your final hip extension range of motion. This is not for you if you have a significant loss of hip extension range of motion.

Position: Lie on the floor with one leg bent at the knee and calf supported on a chair and the other leg out straight on the floor.

Neutral Back: The stretch is aimed at the front of the hip and thigh of the leg that is straight out on the floor. Ideally your back is in the neutral position. However, it might have a slight arch. Do not try to prevent the arch; working to keep your back from arching places too much pressure on your back and pelvis. Do not perform it if arching is a position that increases your pain, or if your pain starts to increase while doing this exercise.

Isolate the Movement: Do not force a stretch. Have your back in its most comfortable position closest to neutral; see Figure 7-19. If you have limited hip extension range of motion, this position should provide a stretch sensation over the front of your hip.

Duration and Repetition: Hold a gentle stretch for 30 seconds, repeat three times.

Exercise (20) Floor Clock Series in Lying Down Position:

The name floor clock is used to identify the varying positions of your arms. Your head is in the 12:00 position, your legs are in the 6:00 position, and the position of your arms varies with each exercise.

Position: Lie on your back on the floor with your hips and knees bent. Your feet can be on the floor or up on a chair. You can have your head on a pillow or on the floor.

Neutral Back: Move your back into the neutral position. If you use the chair, to move into the neutral position you might need to pull the chair close to your hips to bend your hips more and decrease the arch in your back or move the chair towards your feet to decrease the bend at your hips and increase the arch in your back.

Floor Clock A: Chest Stretch

Isolate the Movement: This exercise is aimed at the front of the chest under the collar bone and across the front of the arms, you might not feel a sensation. Place your arms out to the side at a position of 3:00 for the left arm and 9:00 for the right arm. Keep your elbows straight and your palms facing up; see Figure 7-20a. Relax and allow gravity to move your shoulders back, opening up your chest.

Duration and Repetition: Initially hold the stretch for up to five minutes. If your body tolerates this position and you have no increase in pain or symptoms, slowly progress up to 45 minutes.

Floor Clock B: Arms Moving Down Towards 6:00

Isolate the Movement: The affect of this exercise is aimed at the shoulders to help them maintain an upright position while your arms are at your side. There will be minimal to no sensation with this exercise. The first time you are looking to find the best arm position for the exercise. Slide your arms all the way down to your hips in one slow smooth movement. At some point your shoulders will lift up off the floor; keep moving your arms all the way down to your hips. Note the position where your shoulders lift up off the floor, for example, left arm at 4:00 and right arm at 8:00. Start again at 3:00 and 9:00 and slide your arms down, this time stop at the point where your shoulders lifted up the first time. Hold the position there. Do not force your shoulders back, rather let gravity work to open your chest; see Figure 7-20b. You will use the same position for several weeks before you can move your arms further.

Duration and Repetition: Hold that position for up to five minutes.

Floor Clock C: Arms Moving Up Towards 12:00

Isolate the Movement: The stretch is aimed at the outside of your shoulders. Slide your arms up toward 12:00. Stop when you feel the first sensation under your arms; see Figure 7-20c. If you go too far, you will feel the sensation on the top of your shoulders. Stop, reposition, and start again. If you have the shoulder sensation again, stop the exercise and talk with your PT.

Duration and Repetition: Hold a gentle stretch for up to five minutes.

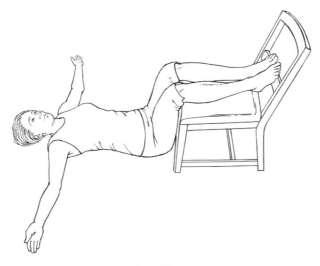

Fig. 7-20a

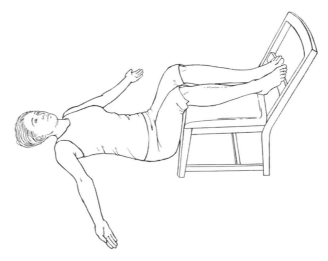

Fig. 7-20b

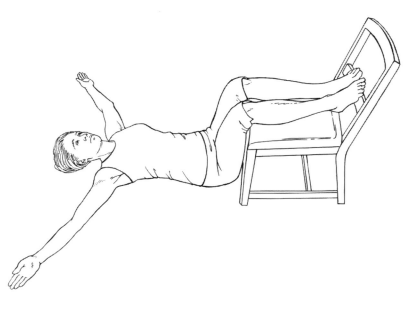

Fig. 7-20c

Arms on Pillows: If in any of the floor clock exercises you have pain either behind or on top of your shoulders, you might not be ready to have your chest open all the way with your arms on the floor. In this case, bring your arms closer to your chest by raising them on pillows. If using one pillow for each arm, place it below the elbow. If using two pillows for each arm, place one above the elbow and the other below the elbow with a towel rolled up under your hand; see Figure 7-20d. You cannot do this exercise if it causes any sensation on the top or back of the shoulders.

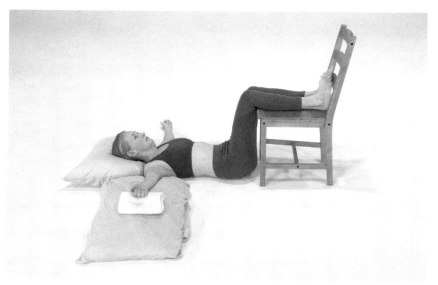

Fig. 7-20d

Exercise (21) Side Neck Stretch

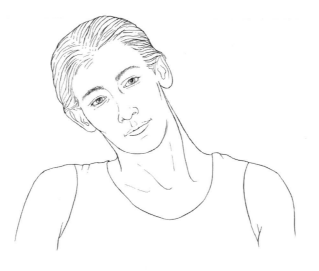

Fig. 7-21

Position: Sitting or standing. Neck in middle or most pain free position.

Neutral Back: Back in neutral or most pain free position.

Isolate the Movement: This stretch is aimed on the side of the neck that is moving away from your shoulder, also known as the side of the neck that is elongating. Tilt your head to the side until you feel the first sensation on the side of your neck; see Figure 21. When moving your head back to upright, tuck your chin slightly to minimize the risk of catching or pinching something in your neck. Stop the exercise if you get a sensation on the side you are leaning towards; something is getting pinched or aggravated. Re-position and try again. Do not do this exercise as long as you continue to have sensation on the side you lean towards.

Duration and Repetition: Hold the stretch for 10 seconds, repeat three times.

Exercise (22) Rear and Side Neck Stretch

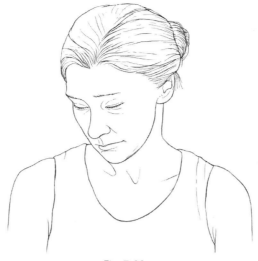

Fig. 7-22

Position: Sitting or standing. Neck in middle or most pain free position.

Neutral Back: Back in neutral or most pain free position.

Isolate the Movement: The stretch is aimed at the side of the back of your neck. Turn you head slightly to one side, drop your chin down until your feel the first sensation on the side you are leaning away from; see Figure 7-22. Slowly return head to upright to minimize chance of catching or pinching any tissue. Stop the exercise if you get a sensation on the side you are turning towards; something is getting pinched or aggravated. Re-position and try again. Do not do this exercise as long as you continue to have sensation on the side you lean towards.

Duration and Repetition: Hold the stretch for 10 seconds, repeat three times.

Exercise (23) Shoulder Retraction

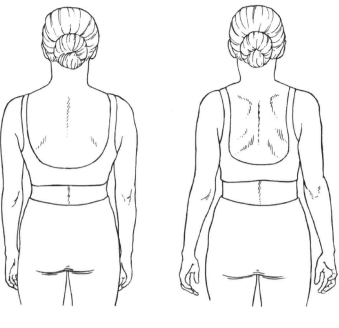

Fig. 7-23a   Fig 7-23b

Position: Sitting or standing.

Neutral Back: Back in neutral or most pain free position.

Isolate the Movement: The exercise is aimed at contracting the muscle between your shoulder blades and possibly a stretch in the front of the chest; see Figure 7-23a. Move the shoulder blades together by contracting muscles between your shoulder blades until you feel a stretch in the front of your chest or until you have contracted your muscles as much as you can; see Figure 7-23b. Do not try so hard that your back arches. When you relax make sure you let the shoulders move all the way back to the standing position.

Duration and Repetition: To stretch chest, hold 20 seconds, repeat three times. To increase muscle control and strength, hold two seconds, repeat 15 times.

MOTOR CONTROL

GENERAL INSTRUCTIONS FOR IMPROVING MOTOR CONTROL

The goal of all trunk stabilization exercises is to improve motor control by keeping your back in the neutral position while moving your arms or legs. For each exercise:

1) Assume the functional position for the exercise (lie down, sit, stand, etc.).
2) Assume the neutral (or most pain-free) back position, contract abdominals to hold position.
3) Start the exercise and maintain the neutral (or most pain-free) back position.
4) Stop the exercise if you lose the neutral (or most pain-free) back position.
5) Work up to performing the exercise for two minutes without losing the neutral (or most pain-free) back position.
6) Once you can perform the exercises for the legs for two minutes, combine the arm and leg exercises into one exercise.

Trunk Stabilization Series in Hook-Lying Position:

For all Trunk Stabilization Exercises in Hook-lying:

Position: Assume the hook-lying position, lie on your back on the floor with your hips and knees bent. Do this on the floor. This exercise is difficult to do on a surface that is soft like a bed.

Neutral Back: Move your back into the neutral position. Contract your abdominals to maintain your back in the neutral position throughout the exercise.

Exercise (25) Hook-Lying: Alternate Leg Lift

Isolate the Movement: Special instructions for hand placement. Although the hand placement will be under your back in the hook-lying position, the hand placement is demonstrated here in standing; see Figure 7-24, Place your hands under your back so that your first knuckle is in contact with the most prominent bone in your pelvis at the base of your spine. This position is done to monitor for back movement in order to make sure the movement is from the hips and not from the back.

Any change of pressure on the hands while you lift a leg means that your back has moved during the activity. Before the exercise note the pressure on both hands. When you start to lift a leg take as much weight off the leg as can WITHOUT any changes in the pressure on your hands. You might only be able to take a couple of pounds off your leg, or just think about lifting the leg, while leaving the rest of the leg in contact with the floor.

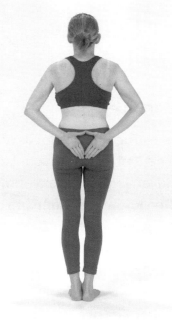

Fig. 7-24

Exercise (25) continued

The focus of the exercise number 25 is to move your legs while you keep your back in neutral. Place your hands as instructed under your back. Move your back into neutral. Contract your abdominal muscles to hold your back in neutral (but not so much that you flattens your back onto the floor). Note the pressure on both hands. The goal is to alternately lift each leg ½ inch off the floor without the pressure changing on your hands; see Figure 7-25. Note if the pressure changes on your hands. If so your back is moving and is not stable. Re-position to the neutral position and this time lift only as much weight off your legs as you can while keeping the pressure the same on both hands. You might only be able to take a couple of pounds off your leg. Start with what you can do WITHOUT the pressure changing on your hands. Over time you will be able to lift more weight off your leg until you can finally lift your foot off the floor. Alternate lifting each leg without moving your back.

> **Duration and Repetition:** Start with alternating five times. Take as long as you need to perform the five repetitions. Perform three sets. Build up to alternating for two minutes, one time.

Exercise (26) Hook-Lying: Arm Lift

> **Isolate the Movement:** As per the instructions the focus of the exercise is to move your arms while you keep your back in neutral. Raise both arms at the same time. Somewhere before you get to shoulder height, your back will start to arch. At that point contract your abdominal muscles to prevent your back from arching and move your arms two or three inches further, if that's possible without your back arching; see Figure 7-26. Then lower your arms back to your side, relax your abdominal muscles at the same point where you contracted them, and continue to lower your arms to the floor. Stop exercise and talk with your PT if you have any shoulder sensation.

> **Duration and Repetition:** Repeat five to six times.

Exercise (27) Hook-Lying: Arm and Leg Lift

> **Isolate the Movement:** As per the instructions the focus of the exercise is to move your arms and legs and keep your back in neutral. Contract your stomach muscles to keep your back in neutral. Raise your right arm and left leg at the same time about two inches off the ground, keeping your back in neutral, then lower your right arm and left leg at the same time. Then lift your left arm and right leg about two inches off the ground, keeping your back in neutral; see Figure 7-27. Keep your back in neutral while repeating the above exercise. When you can, your PT will have you add weights to your hands and ankles.

> **Duration and Repetition:** Initially alternate five times, and do three sets of five each. Build up to performing the exercise for two minutes.

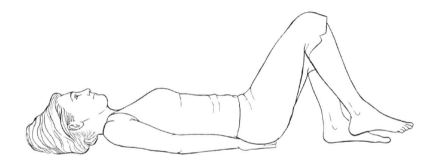

Fig. 7-25

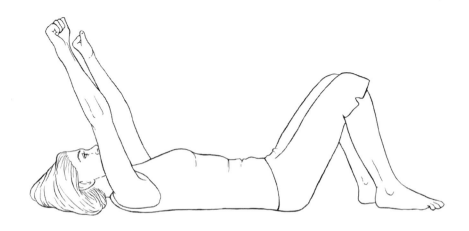

Fig. 7-26

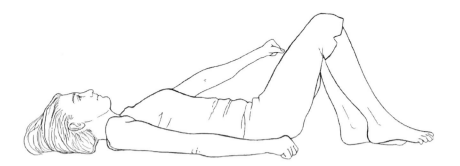

Fig. 7-27

TRUNK STABILIZATION SERIES IN STANDING POSITION:

Exercise (28) Standing: Mini-Squat

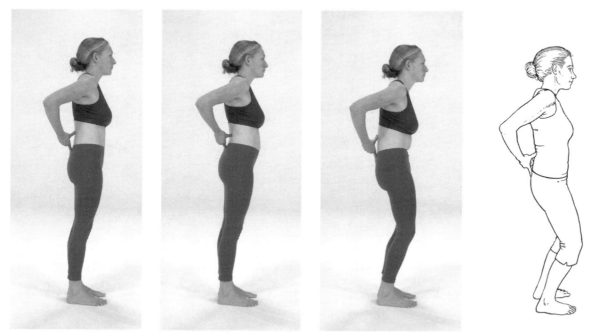

Fig. 7-28a   Fig. 7-28b   Fig. 7-28c   Fig. 28d

Position: Standing.

Neutral Back: Keeping your back in the neutral position is the goal of the exercise. Place a hand on your low back with your first finger on the base of your spine and your thumb three to four inches higher on your spine; see Figure 7-28a. Arch your back and feel your fingers move together; see Figure 7-28b. Move back to the neutral position. Then flatten your back and feel your fingers move apart; see Figure 7-28c. Move back to the neutral position and contract your abdominals to try to maintain the neutral position throughout your exercise. If not held stable your back will tend to flatten when squatting down and arch when returning to upright.

Isolate the Movement: The focus of the exercise is to keep your back in neutral while you perform a slight mini-squat. With your thumb on your spine and your first finger on the base of your spine, bend at your hips and knees into a mini-squat, contract abdominals to help keep your back in neutral; see Figure 7-28d. Come back up to standing. Monitor your back position with your hand.

Duration and Repetition: Do a mini-squat 5-10 times, repeat three sets.

Note: Returning to standing without arching your back requires almost full hip extension range of motion. If you do not have full hip extension range of motion, either you cannot do the exercise at this time or the exercise needs to be modified.

To modify this exercise, start with a slight bend in your hips and knees; see Figure 7-28d. Squat down slightly from that starting position. Then return to the new starting position with your hips and knees bent. You can repeat this three to five times. It will help you learn to control your back position.

Exercise (29) Standing: Arm Lift

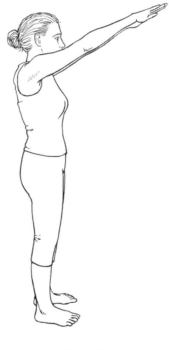

Fig. 7-29

Isolate the Movement: The focus of this exercise is to keep your back in neutral while you raise both arms. Focus on your back staying in the neutral position, contract your abdominals to help maintain your neutral position while you lift both arms up in front of you. Lift them up only as much as you can with your shoulders comfortable, moving no higher than just above shoulder height. Lower your arms back down; see Figure 7-29.

Duration and Repetition: Repeat three to five times. Monitor your shoulders; if they start to have any sensation or pain during or after the exercise, stop this exercise and talk to your PT.

Exercise (30) Standing: Mini-Squat with Arm Lift

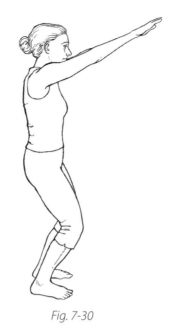

Fig. 7-30

Isolate the Movement: The focus of this exercise is to keep your back in neutral while you perform a mini-squat and raise both arms. Focus on your back staying in the neutral position, contract your abdominals to keep your back in neutral. Move from standing into a slight mini-squat while lifting both your arms up in front of you; see Figure 7-30. Return to standing while lowering arms to your side.

Duration and Repetition: Start with five repetitions. Increase up to two minutes.

Strength

GENERAL INSTRUCTIONS FOR STRENGTHENING EXERCISES

- Your exercises are selected to address areas of decreased strength from your list of mechanical limitations. If you do not yet tolerate a manual muscle test your PT will decide which areas to address based on factors that indicate areas of decreased strength.

Exercise technique is important for effectiveness. We need research to determine the most effective exercises to strengthen. Meanwhile, keep the following points in mind while you develop each of your exercises:

- Remember to always move your back into the neutral position before starting the exercise, and contract your abdominal muscles to help maintain the neutral position throughout the exercise.
- Focus your movement on the muscle to be strengthened.
- Keep the movement within your available range of motion and within your muscle's ability to perform the exercise; otherwise you might pull your back out of its neutral or most pain free position to help perform the exercise.

When you are building your program also keep in mind the following:

- Train your muscles in the manner in which they function.
  Postural muscles contract at a low level for a long period for time. Exercise 31, the Prone Retraction Series, is an example of strengthening with a low level contraction, building up to a prolonged period of time. For postural stability you want to strengthen the muscles in your upper back that are designed to contract at a low level for a long period of time.
  Power muscles produce a forceful contraction for a short duration. Exercise 32, the Hip Abduction exercise, is an example of a strengthening exercise held for a short duration. Many of you with back pain will not be using heavy weights and performing forceful contractions; however, typically heavy weight and a short contraction time are used to strengthen power muscles.
- Use Pain as your guide.

When you work on developing your exercises, some exercises might increase your pain. Work with your PT to make the necessary adjustments. The goal is to develop exercises that never increase your pain, and to find some that decrease your pain.

Exercise (31) Prone Retraction Series, for Upper Body Strengthening

For all prone exercises:

Position: Lie on your stomach with pillows for positioning.

Neutral Back: Position pillows to help you easily get in and stay in the neutral position. Your neck should be comfortable and in the middle position, not arched backward or rounded forward. You and your PT need to work with the thickness of the pillows and towel roll to accomplish a good position for your neck and back. You might use one pillow with its length from your shoulder to your hips and another pillow cross-wise under your hips. If your head tends to be forward of your shoulders, to create a comfortable position you might place both pillows length wise from your shoulders to your hips. Place a towel roll under your forehead, to create a place for your nose. Move your back into neutral. Contract your abdominals to help maintain your back in the neutral position throughout the exercise.

Prone Retraction A: Prone Retraction

Isolate the Movement: The exercise is aimed at strengthening the muscles between the shoulder blades. Squeeze your shoulder blades together moving towards your spine; see Figure 7-31a. Focus on the contraction of the muscles between your shoulder blades. Do not go so far that you arch your back. The only sensation should be between your shoulder blades, not in your neck or low back. If you feel something in your neck or low back, stop the exercise and review it again with your PT.

Duration and Repetition: Hold for two seconds, repeat ten times.

Prone Retraction B: Arm Lift

Isolate the Movement: The exercise is aimed at strengthening the muscles between the shoulder blades. Squeeze your shoulder blades together as in Prone retraction A, then lift your arms ½ inch off the floor; see Figure 7-31b. You should feel the sensation only between your shoulder blades, not in your neck or low back. Relax by putting your arms down and then your shoulder blades.

Duration and Repetition: Squeeze your shoulder blades together, lift your arms 1 inch, hold two seconds, then relax back down. Repeat ten times.

Prone Retraction C: Head Lift

Neutral Back: Position the pillows to help you into the neutral position. This exercise includes steps to assure that you maximally contract your abdominals to try to prevent your back from arching.

Isolate the Movement: The exercise is aimed at strengthening the muscles between the shoulder blades and increasing shoulder girdle stability. Performing this exercise takes four steps: 1) tighten your stomach muscles and tuck your bottom under slightly to minimize the chance of your back arching, 2) move your shoulder blades together, 3) check your abdominal muscles to make sure they are fully contracting, and 4) Lift your head ¼ inch off the towel roll. Your head should lift straight up so that you are still looking down; see Figure 7-31c. Do not arch your neck up by lifting your chin up, and do not bend your neck down by tucking your chin in. The sensation should be between your shoulder blades and not in your neck or back.

Duration and Repetition: Initially hold for five seconds, and repeat five times. Work up to holding the head lift for 30 seconds, and repeat three times.

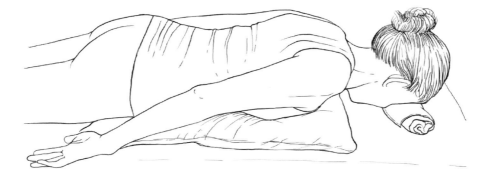

Fig. 7-31a

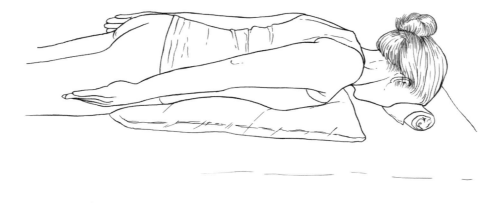

Fig. 7-31b

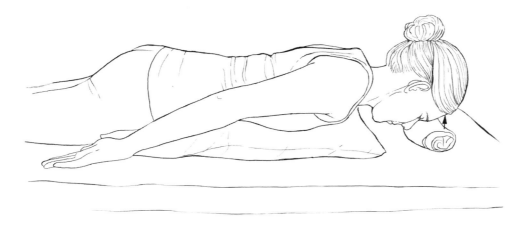

Fig. 7-31c

Exercise (32) Hip Abduction Strengthening

Position: Lie on your side. Position your body as straight as you can. You can bend the bottom leg for balance. Place the upper arm on the floor or mat for balance. Position the arm underneath so it is comfortable. In this exercise your body can tend to roll backwards and bend at the hip in order to use the muscles on the front of your leg. Try to prevent both by slightly rolling your body forward.

Neutral Back: Position your back in neutral, not arched or flattened. Also position your back in neutral and not bent to the side. If your waist is smaller than your hips or shoulders, place a small pillow under your waist to help keep your back in neutral. Contract your abdominals to hold your back in neutral.

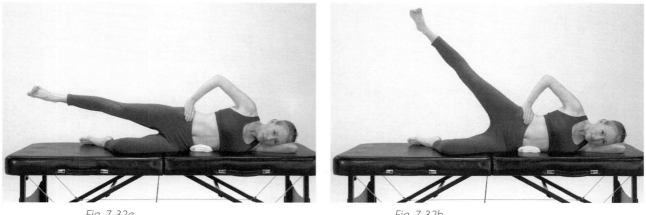

Fig. 7-32a   Fig. 7-32b

Isolate the Movement: The muscle you are trying to strengthen is over your hip, at the side of your bottom, just behind where the seam of your pant's run down. The work should be felt in that area. Raise your upper leg toward the ceiling; see Figure 7-32a. Focus on moving only from the hip joint, not from the back. Feel the sensation of work only over your hip just behind the seam of your pants. Do not bend at your hip or roll you hip backwards. Slowly lower your leg down, keeping your back in neutral.

Do not go beyond your hip's available range of motion, because that would cause movement from your back to help get the leg to the higher position. Note in Figure 7-32b that her hand and rib cage are closer together. This demonstrates that her back has bent to the side. The back moved to help lift her leg higher. In Figure 7-32a she only moved her leg as far as the hip joint could move it and her back stayed in the neutral position. You can monitor for back movement by making sure your hand/hip do not move. Raise your leg up toward the ceiling only as far as you can without your hand moving.

Duration and Repetition: Hold two seconds and relax. Repeat ten times.

CHAPTER 8

Challenges in Treatment

CHALLENGES IN CURRENT TREATMENT OF BACK PAIN

THERE are numerous challenges in the current treatment of back pain. The anatomy, the location, and the job of the spine all present a challenge. Everyone involved in the treatment of back pain—the clinicians, the health care system, the patients, the insurance industry, etc.—all contribute their own unique challenges to the treatment of back pain. Before starting my own clinic, I worked as a traveling physical therapist and locally as a temporary physical therapist, which gave me the opportunity to work in more than 40 clinics, including hospitals, outpatient offices, rehabilitation hospitals, and long term care facilities. Following are my observations.

Keep in mind that these challenges, not present in every clinic, are my observations and opinions. I believe these are some of the issues that can effect the treatment of your back pain.

KNOWLEDGE OF WHAT TO TREAT: THE CAUSE OR THE SYMPTOM

Knowledge of what to treat is the most significant challenge in the treatment of back pain. When the cause of back pain is unknown 85 percent of the time,[14] knowing what to treat is clearly a problem. This leads to a subsequent challenge, which is that many people agree to treat their pain as an acceptable replacement for treating the underlying problem. If you had a broken bone or a heart attack you would not consider treating the pain as an acceptable replacement for treating the problem. You might be pleased with attention to the pain but most of you would want the primary focus to be on the evaluation and treatment of the underlying cause of the pain, the heart attack or the broken bone. I think we need this for back pain too: to not accept treating pain as a replacement for treating the underlying cause of the back pain.

RECURRENCE

Recurrence is pain that comes back after it has disappeared for a period of time. The question that needs to be answered is, when the pain goes away is the underlying problem resolved? Finding an answer to this question is important because it impacts the decisions of people who treat back pain, people who have back pain, and the people who pay for the treatment of back pain.

A claim you might find in some resources about back pain is that 90 percent of the time back pain resolves in one month. This claim raises the questions:

- Does this mean the pain is resolved forever?
- Or is the claim misleading? Are the underlying problems still there while the pain has only subsided for a temporary period of time?

A study in 1998 investigating that claim found that only 25 percent recovered completely after 12 months.[15]

In another study one conclusion was that pain is less persistent in younger people.[16] My perspective is that older people are just the younger people who haven't had the underlying problem addressed, so over time their back wears down and the pain starts to come on more frequently and for longer periods of time.

FINANCIAL

The subject of financial challenges in health care is a book in itself. Many people can't afford medical help, and for those who can, the financial issues negatively influence many aspects of their care. A major influence is the emphasis on productivity in the clinic. Productivity in this sense does not refer to how productive the clinician is in alleviating the patient's problems. Rather, it refers to financial productivity, meaning the number of patients seen and the amount billed. Businesses do need to have a financial plan. However, when financial productivity is the driving force behind the daily schedule and the hour-to-hour decisions about the schedule, it is difficult to keep effective treatment of the patient as the main focus.

In 1998 the U.S. spent $90.1 billion on back pain, including 27.9 billion on inpatient care, 23.6 billion on offices visits, 14.1 billion on prescription drugs, 11.9 billion on outpatient services, 2.7 billion on emergency room visits, and 2.7 billion on home health services.[17] It seems that there is a lot of money being spent, so the question might be, is it being spent to most effectively treat patients?

When I started my practice I decided not to participate with any insurance companies. I felt in the past that it made it very difficult to get my work done. I found the paper work time consuming and distracting as well as finding it disruptive to treatment to constantly rely on a third party who is not present to make decisions about the person's ability to attend treatment.

However, on behalf of one of my patients, I once submitted an appeal to an insurance company. The insurance company had denied payment for any further physical therapy and in my opinion the therapy was reasonable and necessary. In short, she had made tremendous progress however she had much more progress to make. At the time of the denial the patient was still having days where she would have to lie down in the back seat of the car in order to get to work. The complaint was reviewed at multiple levels and each professional reviewer supported the original insurance company denial. The complaint worked its way up to the court of appeals. The judge found in our favor and wrote a 23 page opinion in which she enumerated the faults of the insurance company. It was nice to have someone validate my complaint, however, my real concern is how could multiple levels of professionals make the same erroneous conclusion when I was working so hard to inform them otherwise.

CLINICIANS

Clinicians find themselves in the middle of all the challenges in health care. As discussed in Chapter 4, under finding a physical therapist, there are multiple challenges for PTs. Challenges include treating numerous disorders, having inadequate time to see patients and having multiple therapists treat the same patient. There is also tremendous paperwork demands: the clinic's paperwork, the licensure requirements, and countless different insurance requirements. There are goals to address, all with different timing. Tracking the true progress of the patient can present with very different timing day to day or week to week than is requested by the PT licensure requirements and the insurance company requirements. Getting the day's work done can be a challenge, therefore learning new treatments and keeping up on new research can seem impossible.

In some cases the PT only has time to do certain tests during an evaluation even if the PT's desire is to do more. Without the tests the PT does not know what information they are missing about the patient's body. Of course a significant challenge for all clinicians treating back pain is knowledge of what to treat, as that has been an issue for all clinicians treating back pain.

HEALTH CARE SYSTEM

In my experience many clinicians enter into a system in which they have little control. It seems that the paperwork and the productivity pressures have the greatest control over their time. In some clinics where I worked I felt like the clinicians were supporting the system instead of the system supporting the work of the clinicians.

Most clinics are not set up to easily allow the clinician to respond to individual patient needs and schedule time with the patient as the clinician deems necessary. If the clinician does not have time for an adequate evaluation of the problem, it is a challenge to develop an effective treatment program. If productivity meant productive results for the patients, the needs of each patient would determine the schedule and a system would be in place for the PT to easily schedule time with the patient according to his or her needs. Unfortunately, productivity in most cases means financial productivity.

Paperwork is a huge issue that challenges the clinician and impacts the treatment. Paperwork takes much of the clinician's time away from the patient. Most clinicians do not get reimbursed for that time.

PATIENTS

Following are a number of patient challenges:

Cost: Many people cannot afford the treatment.

Difficult choices: Many people want to get better but unfortunately have multiple serious demands on their time that compete with their ability to follow through with treatment programs.

Forget original pain: The most common issue I see in the clinic is that patients forget their original pain. The challenge here is that if they do not realize their progress, they cannot learn what they did to decrease the original pain. Failing to learn what they did to decrease their pain is a huge loss to their ability to further progress. This also presents a challenge if the clinician does not have a measurable record of the original pain. The clinician might change a program that is effective because the patient does not see improvement.

Quick fix: Many people are looking for a quick fix. Even when they intellectually realize that it takes time to properly address a problem, emotionally they want immediate gratification. I often draw the analogy to weight loss. Although someone might want to lose 50 pounds in a month, most of us realize that doing it quickly is not a good idea for their health and the results do not last long.

Expectations: Patients who expect a complete recovery and a swift return to their previous levels of activity generally do not grasp the condition in which they arrived for treatment and the significance of the history of warning signs.

HOW THIS APPROACH ADDRESSES THE CHALLENGES

Following is how the System Limitations Approach to Pain can help address some of the challenges outlined in the previous section.

KNOWLEDGE OF WHAT TO TREAT: THE CAUSE OR THE SYMPTOM

In this approach the evaluation focuses on identifying mechanical limitations that *cause* your back pain. The mechanical limitations identified as the *cause* then become the focus of your treatment.

If mechanical limitations are the *cause* of your back pain, your pain and symptoms are expected to decrease as a result of focusing the treatment on the cause.

It will be interesting to find out how many of the 85 percent of those with non-specific low back pain are identified as having mechanical limitations as the cause of their pain.

RECURRENCE

For those of you who have mechanical limitations causing your back pain, I believe that addressing the underlying problem will decrease your pain's recurrence and persistence.

For most of you with mechanical limitations, the pain came on with increasing frequency and intensity and it will go out in the reverse, with episodes of decreasing frequency and intensity. It will not just go away tomorrow. Research is needed before we can forecast how far you will progress given your unique set of limitations.

FINANCIAL

This approach will increase the amount of time and money you spend with a PT *in the beginning* because the evaluation and initial sessions take longer and require one-on-one time with the PT. You will also be supervised by the PT for a much longer period of time.

I am convinced that *in the long run* this approach saves money for the treatment of those with mechanical limitations that cause their pain. The decrease in the cost of back pain treatment is in part because: 1) addressing the underlying problem should decrease the intensity, duration, and recurrence of your back pain, 2) you do most of your treatment program at home, 3) you learn ways to manage your pain and ways to decrease your pain on your own, and 4) successful treatment decreases the need for visits to numerous different health care clinicians now and down the road.

In clinics where the primary focus is on financial productivity, the hope is that this approach will be the great equalizer. I believe this approach will demonstrate better results, and so those who pay for care will seek physical therapists who provide this approach to back pain for patients with mechanical limitations that cause their pain.

Regarding those who cannot afford care, I hope that research and feedback from multiple clinics might help us learn how to best organize care for those who do not have the resources or who live in areas that are underserved.

CLINICIANS

This approach addresses a number of challenges. It uses certain basic measurements that every PT learned in school so there is not the concern of having to learn some unfamiliar information. What's new in this approach, as distinct from what has been learned in school, is about measurements; helping the patient report his or her pain in measurable terms, using measurement techniques to increase the probability that the results reflect the intended measurement and taking measurements throughout the body that could impact the back.

This approach works to address the underlying cause of back pain, advocates for adequate time for evaluation and treatment, and uses objective data for developing treatment plans and assessing progress. This should be helpful in keeping the program and patient on track.

Two challenges remain for the clinician:

1) The theory is simple, but developing a program for a complex body in a complex life in some cases can be quite challenging.
2) Research is needed to identify the most effective and efficient means to improve overall mechanics in the human body.

HEALTH CARE SYSTEM

In a perfect world the clinician would understand what needs to be done, the patient would follow through with the program, and the health care system would facilitate a clinical setup that supports the clinician and the patient. However, this is not a perfect world. The health care system has a structure and expectations that are difficult for individual therapists to change. Fortunately the SLAP approach is based on obtaining detailed, objective and measurable information. The hope is that with the measurable data and the clear relationship between the pain and limitations, this approach will facilitate a change in the present structure of how treatment for back pain is delivered.

Consider this example of a problem and a possible solution:

> The accepted structure in the health care system puts each patient in a time slot of 45 to 60 minutes for a physical therapy evaluation, regardless of the complexity of the patient's problem. The follow-up sessions are routinely set for 2-3 times a week in a predetermined time slot that again, does not consider the intensity of the patient's problem. Meanwhile, during the treatment session the PT manages multiple patients at one time, resulting in some cases in less than 20 minutes with each patient. The PT's attention is often divided between patients.

> A more effective structure would allow the time for the evaluation to be completed. I find that, on average, a three-hour time slot is needed to gather the measurements about both the patient's mechanics and about his or her pain. I have tried to gather the information over three one-hour sessions and have found it difficult to obtain the big picture; the information

becomes disorganized for both the patient and I. Once the PT has the information in an organized big picture, s/he better understands the patient's mechanical system. A better assessment paves the way for a more effective program.

The follow-up sessions focus on the patient learning to manage the pain and on developing a customized exercise program. This requires focused one-on-one time with the same PT each session. The patient learns how to independently manage his or her pain 24 hours a day, 7 days a week. In the beginning the sessions are longer and more frequent than typically scheduled for treatment sessions. Eventually the time pays off because the PT better understands the patient mechanically. The program is customized for the patient's problems. In the present structure the patient can learn in a few weeks what previously would have taken much longer to accomplish. The patient does most of the work at home.

The more intense initial sessions could decrease use of pain medication, decrease lost time at work, and decrease emergency visits to the doctor for pain relief, to name a few advantages. This structure could be more productive for the patient and more financially productive overall.

PATIENTS

Cost: The SLAP approach should ultimately decrease the cost of treating back pain in the population as a whole. The question is whether the funds that are saved will then be made available to take care of those who cannot afford care.

Difficult choices: Patients use many aspects of this program during their everyday activities, rather than in competition with life's other demands. Developing and following the exercise program does take time; hopefully the patients' ability to decrease their own pain helps relieve some of the burden of performing life's activities for those whose lives are demanding.

Forget Original Pain: The detailed evaluation helps many patients identify the cause of their pain, as well as remember their original pain so that they can learn to decrease their own pain and gain control over their bodies.

Quick Fix: This does not help people who want a quick fix. Hopefully after the evaluation, patients will understand that a quick fix is not the answer

Patient Expectations: Knowledge is a powerful thing. One hopes that when patients see and feel the limitations in their bodies they will have a better understanding of what they need to do, what they can do, and what the PT can and cannot do for them.

When people understand their limitations, they are better able to make decisions about how to decrease their pain while at work, at home, and at social events. This allows them to have more control, increasing the quality of their life. This control impacts many serious aspects of patients' lives, including their relationships, level of independence, and ability to perform daily responsibilities.

APPENDIX A

Glossary of Terms

WEBSTER New World Dictionary of the American Language (2d College Ed. 1986), (used as a reference for defining terms)

Abduction: To move away from the side of the body.

Activities of Daily Living (ADL): Activities that you do each day, for example dressing, bathing, and grooming.

Acute: Historically referred to pain of less than 30 days' duration; however, now can also refer to severe pain rather than just the time frame.

Adduction: To move toward the center of the body.

Ankle Dorsiflexion: Joint movement of the ankle that moves the foot up towards the front of the body.

Anterior Superior Iliac Spine (ASIS): boney prominence on the front of the pelvis.

Arch: 1. the area on the bottom of your foot that is raised up between the heel and the toes; 2. the position of the low back where there is a concave curvature; 3. the action of moving the back into a curved position.

Bend: Move a joint from a straightened or angular position to a more angular position.

Big Four Mechanics: The four main tools the human body uses to produce movement and to move into specific stationary positions, such as sitting, standing, or lying down.

Big Four Mechanical Limitations: Restriction of the tools the human body uses to produce movement or achieve stationary positions such as sitting, standing, or lying down.

Calcaneal Eversion: A movement of the ankle in which the bottom of the heel moves out to the side away from the body.

Chronic: Lasting a long time or recurring.

Contraindication: A matter, circumstance or health problem that makes treatment inadvisable.

Deep Postural Muscles: Muscles that lie close to the skeleton, that contract in a manner to provide static control of the body rather than powerful movement of the body.

Dorsiflexion: Movement of the ankle that moves the foot up towards the nose.

Evaluation: In this context, a procedure to determine the condition of the human body mechanics in relation to pain.

Evaluation of Mechanical Limitations: See Evaluation.

Extend: To move a body part towards the straightened position.

Extension: 1. the joint position in which the joint is straight; or 2. the action of moving the joint to a straight position.

Flatten: Movement of the lower spine backwards out of the arched position to a more flat position.

Flex: Moving a joint from a straightened position to a bent position.

Flexion: 1. the joint position in which the joint is bent; or 2. the action of moving the joint to a bent position.

Functional Position: Positions the body moves into to perform daily activities. Examples are sitting, standing, and lying down.

Hip Abduction: Movement of the hip joint that moves the leg out to the side away from the side of the body.

Hip Adduction: Hip joint movement that moves the leg in towards the center of the body.

Hip External Rotation: Hip joint movement that rolls the leg out.

Hip Flexion: Hip joint movement that bends the leg towards the stomach.

Hip Internal Rotation: Hip joint movement that rolls the leg in.

Manual Muscle Test (MMT): Procedure to identify how strong muscles are.

Mechanics: The body's tools that are involved in producing dynamic and static activity.

Mechanical Limitations: In this context, restriction in the tools the human body uses for movement and to achieve a stationary position.

Motor Control: The tool the brain uses to control and coordinate the body.

Neutral Spine: Position of the spine and pelvis in which the forces on the body are distributed most economically. Generally defined as the position where the ASIS and PSIS are in the same plane; in a standing position that plane would be parallel with the floor.

Pelvis: Large circular bone positioned between the spine and the leg.

Physical Therapist (PT): Licensed professional who attended and graduated from an accredited school of physical therapy.

Posterior Superior Iliac Spine (PSIS): boney prominence on the back of the pelvis.

Postural Alignment: In general how the human body lines up in standing, more specifically, how each part of the body relates to each other when standing upright.

Range of Motion: The distance through which a joint can move.

Rotate: Turning of a joint right or left, or in or out.

Shoulder Girdle: The area in the upper back that the arms attach to.

Specific Position: An exact position of the back. The specific position of the low back can be arched, slightly arched, neutral, slightly flattened, flattened, rotated right, rotated left, bent to the right side, or bent to the left side.

Stabilization: In the context of this book, the ability to keep the back position from changing or fluctuating.

Strength: Force generated by muscle activity.

Thoracic: The name for the area of the upper two thirds of the back.

Trunk: The term for the body not including the head, arms, or legs.

Trunk Stabilization: The ability to keep the trunk position from changing or fluctuating.

Vertebrae: The individual bones that make up the spine.

Vertebral Body: The large circular bone on the front of the vertebrae.

Following are the abbreviations I use in this book and what they stand for:

ADL: Activities of Daily Living

ASIS: Anterior Superior Iliac Spine

MMT: Manual Muscle Test

PSIS: Posterior Superior Iliac Spine

PT: Physical Therapist

ROM: Range of Motion

Research

RESEARCH plays a vital role in health care. Research helps us understand what the tests really measure and whether the treatment has the effect we would like it to have. I believe research should play a prominent role in the development of back pain treatment. I struggled with how to handle research in this book, inserting research into each topic in the book would have created a much more complicated book then was my mission or vision. I decided to address the overall topic of research in this section. Following are recent reviews of research about back pain, recommendations for future research, and my opinion of the challenges we face with research on back pain.

Reviews

There have been several reviews of the research on low back pain (LBP). Following is a brief discussion about two publications.

The Diagnosis and Treatment of Low Back Pain: A Joint Clinical Practice Guideline from the American College of Physicians and the American Pain Society, was published in October 2007. This publication suggested that when evaluating the cause of pain that illnesses outside the back should be considered, such as, illnesses of the heart, kidney, or pancreas, as well as systemic illness. It also recommended considering psychological factors.[18] There was no mention of looking outside the back for mechanical limitations.

In 2008, the Orthopedic Section of the American Physical Therapy Association, (APTA) published a continuing education course for physical therapists, Low Back Pain and the Evidence for Effectiveness of Physical Therapy Interventions. Most of the topics addressed evaluation and treatment of back pain aimed directly at the back itself. However, John Jefferson, PT, MSc, COMT, recommended that in cases of "no clearly identifiable source of pain," that, "a more functional assessment may be needed including looking at the connections between the trunk and the periphery."[19] This is the direction I believe we need to head in for both practice and research.

This publication also discusses that, "Although a link between lower extremity flexibility and LBP is often assumed, research has not shown this to be the case."[20] A specific example followed; "No evidence currently exists linking improved hamstring flexibility with improvements in pain and disability among patients with low back pain." [21]

How research is interpreted, and the contribution that specific research like that example can make, is what I hope this book can influence. From the perspective of SLAP, your back would tolerate one limitation such as, hamstring flexibility. I find, in most cases of back pain, that the patient has numerous limitations of which hamstring flexibility is often one, and so improving one problem like hamstring flexibility might help a little, but I would not expect a significant improvement without addressing the numerous other limitations.

Research Recommendations

Following are some of my recommendations of areas that need more research:

1. Basic tests of range of motion, strength, motor control and posture to validate and refine the measurement techniques.
2. The connection between the back and the periphery, more specifically the relationships among the three main points relating limitations and back pain:

    - the relationship between mechanical limitations and the positions of the back that increase pain;
    - the relationship between the positions of the back that increase and decrease pain and the daily activities that increase and decrease pain;
    - the relationship between mechanical limitations and the daily activities that increase and decrease pain.

4. Exercise programs that effectively improve range of motion, strength, postural alignment, and trunk stabilization.
5. How improvements in mechanics can best carry over to daily life, including decreased pain and increased ability to perform activities.
6. Whether improvements in mechanics result in improvements in the spine on film (MRI, x-ray), after several years.

Challenges in research

Research in the area of back pain faces a number of challenges:

1) The Randomized Control Trial (RCT) is the gold standard in research. When a study is described as an RCT, it means that the study was designed to increase the chance that the conclusion of the study is true. That is really important, and thankfully people have worked hard to define the factors needed for a good study.

The challenge the RCT presents in the study of back pain is that it is very controlled, looking at only a few factors in a given set of circumstances. On the other hand the reality of back pain for you and the clinician is that it is multifaceted with numerous lifestyle issues. Essentially research looks at a couple narrowly defined problems at one time while clinically most of you are dealing with numerous broad problems. The RCT is needed; it will take a great deal of coordination and communication to organize studies to build upon each other in order to have technically good studies while working towards meaningful information for you and the clinician to put together your big picture and have it based on research.

I suggested in Chapter 6, Finishing with Your PT, that if you have mechanical limitations that have not been resolved, you should know what they are. Then keep an eye on the research, with the understanding that one study is a small piece of information in the picture of your back pain. Work with a physical therapist to understand what any one study means to you.

2) I once heard a speaker say that any treatment that is not researched based is unethical. I raise this issue not to question whether research is important, it is important. Rather to raise concern about invalidating treatment that has not been researched. In the past decade the importance of research has gained a lot of attention; however, I believe the pendulum has swung too far. Clearly it is difficult to argue that treatment has been effectively studied when only 15 percent of the cause has been diagnosed: that is putting the cart before the horse. Meanwhile there are a lot of people in pain today. As we acknowledge the importance of research, let's be careful to stay open to the possibility that the most effective treatment might be available, however, it might be something that has not yet been selected to be researched.

3) Studies cost money and the money can be hard to find. To give grants for research, many institutions prefer or require that the professional is a full time researcher. Some researchers say this removes them from the clinic where they felt they had a greater sense of what questions to study. Meanwhile, in most settings clinicians do not have the time, financial support, or facilities to run studies. A better connection is needed so that clinicians can provide more input into questions to study; and researchers have a way to more effectively help clinicians understand the studies' implications, and apply the information in practice.

APPENDIX C

The Rescue Your Back Website

WE have a website you can visit at www.RescueYourBack.com.

The primary mission of the book and website is to increase awareness that there is an alternative approach to explore about back pain. The goal is to reach those who have the back and body problems that this approach can help to address.

Initially the Website will include:

- Order page for purchasing the book
- Sample pages of the book
- A blog with area for comments
- List of PT's who offer this approach
- Information page for PT's including courses and PT DVD

How the website will evolve will be based on need and interest. If there is a manageable response, I will try to respond to your questions and remarks individually.

If there is a huge response, we will organize and determine the best way to progress given the need.

APPENDIX D

Contacts For Book Production Sources

Publisher: The Mahon Group, LLC
                    1610 West Street
                    Suite 103
                    Annapolis, MD 21401
                    Telephone: 410-263-0333
                    www.TheMahonGroup.com

Editors: Elana Kann
                    Member, Editorial Freelancers Association
                    Email: ekann@bellsouth.net
                    Website: www.elanakannedit.com

                    Ron Kenner
                    Email: ron@rkedit.com
                    Website: www.rkedit.com

Photographer: Frederick Soo
                    Email: Fred@fredsoo.com
                    Website: www.fredsoo.com

Cover Designer: Elizabeth Tomlin, Graphic Designer
                    Email: elizabethtomlin@live.com

Layout Designer: Jonathan Gullery
                    Books Just Books
                    Website: www.booksjustbooks.com

DVD Production: E. Eric Johnson, III, Producer/Director
                    Lill Monster Motion Pictures
                    Website: www.lillmonster.net

Endnotes

1 Chou R, Qaseem A, Snow V, et al. Diagnoses and Treatment of Low Back Pain: A Joint Clinical Practice Guideline from the American College of Physicians and the American Pain Society. Ann Intern Med. 2007;147:479.

2 Id.

3 Bigos SJ, Holland J, Holland C, Websster JS, Battie M, Malmgren JA. High-quality controlled trials on preventing episodes of back problems: systematic literature review in working-age adults. Spine J. 2009;9:163.

4 Hansson T, Hansson E, Malchau H. Utility of spine surgery: a comparison of common elective orthopaedic surgical procedures. Spine. 2008;33(25):2819.

5 Friedly J, Chan L, Deyo R. Increases in Lumbosacral Injections in the Medicare Population: 1994 to 2001. Spine. 2007;32(16):1754-60.

6 Deyo RA, Mirza SK, Turner JA, Martin BI. Overtreating Chronic Back Pain: Time to Back Off? J Am Board Fam Med. 2009; 22:63.

7 Deyo R, Gray D, Kreuter W. United States Trends in Lumbar Fusion Surgery for Degenerative Conditions. Spine; 30(12):1441.

8 Deyo RA, supra note 6 , at 62.

9 Social Security Administration Office of Policy. Annual Statistical Report on the Social Security Disability Insurance Program, 2005. SSA publication no. 13-11826. Washington, DC: Social Security Administration; 2006.

10 Chou R, supra note 1, at 479.

11 Boulay, C et al. Sagittal alignment of spine and pelvis regulated by pelvic incidence: standard values and prediction of lordosis. Eur Spine J. 2006;15:415-422.

12 Boulay C, supra note 11, at 420.

13 Boulay C, supra note 11, at 420.

14 Chou R, supra note 1, at 479.

15 Croft PR, McFarlane GJ, Papageorgiou AC, Thomas E, Silman AJ. Outcome of low back pain in general practice: a prospective study. *BMJ*. 1998; 316: 1356-9.

16 Cassidy JD, Cote P, Carroll LJ, Kristman V. Incidence and course of low back pain episodes in the general population. *Spine*. 2005; 30: 2817-23.

17 Luo X, Pietrobon R, Sun S, Liu G, Hey L. Estimates and Patterns of Direct Health Care Expenditures Among Individuals With Back Pain in the United States. Spine. 2003;29(1):81.

18 Chou R, supra note 1, at 479.

19 Reprinted with permission from Author, Jefferson J. Lumbar Examination and Assessment. Independent Study Course 18.1.3, Low Back Pain and the Evidence for Effectiveness of Physical Therapy Interventions. La Crosse, WI; 2008:39. Orthopaedic Section, APTA, Inc.

20 Reprinted with permission from Author,Fritz JM, Cleland JA. Low Back Treatment-based Classifications Independent Study Course 18.1.5, Low Back Pain and the Evidence for Effectiveness of Physical Therapy Interventions. La Crosse, WI;2008:19. Orthopaedic Section, APTA, Inc.

21 Id.